Tidbits For Young Doctors And Their Patients

(Journal of a Country Doctor, Part II)

By Donald L. Martin, M.D.

Fairway Press
Lima, Ohio

Table of Contents

Part One: Stories About Perry County, Kentucky

Part Two: Medical Stories And Health Care Issues

Part Three:
Essays On The Current Social Scene

Part Four: Religious Matters And All That

Part Five: Stories From The Long Ago

Introduction

Three years ago I was head over heels involved in getting my first book published, and that was an exciting time. *Referees, Docs And God* (Journal Of A Country Doctor) took about one year to write. I ordered 2,000 books and within a short period of time 1,000 books were sold. My publisher, Fairway Press of Lima, Ohio, told me that I had a rocket take-off and had set an all time record for a new author. The response was certainly beyond my hopes and expectations and I got carried away and ordered 4,000 more. A little over two years later there are 1,000 books left. It was up to me to do much of the marketing and I did this with pleasure. At Old Settler's Week in Salem, Indiana, I had a booth and sold out my supply quickly. At the Black Gold Festival at Hazard, Kentucky, I also had a booth and sold close to 400 books. Perhaps the best part of the trip to Hazard was to meet so many of my former patients and friends and have a wonderful time visiting together.

Because I had written about a number of controversial subjects, not everyone was pleased with my stance and my conclusions. I expected this but the positive elements of the experience of writing the book were far greater than the negative ones. I was given 10 minutes of exposure on Louisville Television Station WAVE at the morning sunrise talk show. I was given publicity in local newspapers and in the *Courier Journal* of Louisville, Kentucky. A number of patients have come to see me as a physician because of my frankness in discussing some of my own personal health problems and this has made it easier for them to talk about things that normally are difficult to discuss.

In this present book titled *Tidbits For Young Doctors And Their Patients*, I have attempted to pass on some information gleaned from 45 years of medical practice. There are many things that one learns after school is over and I hope my contribution is worth the effort I have put into it. For most of us, writing a book is a way to have lots of fun and a new experience.

And, finally, may I ask the reader's indulgence in a habit that I have which is not always appreciated. On issues that I am passionate about, I tend to repeat myself and tell it again. If you encounter this as you read, deal with it as you wish.

Part One:

Stories About Perry County Kentucky

—1— Perry County, Kentucky

"She's Blue, Doc, Come Quick!"

Those words pierced my ears at 2 a.m. as I answered the telephone. I slept in my scrubs and I was ready to go as soon as I pulled off the covers and put on my shoes. I ran the 50 yards from my house to the hospital into the back hallway and into Peggy's room. The nurse was waiting with the tracheotomy set on the bedside table. One look at Peggy told me the story. Her airway was obstructed and she was struggling for air. Her face was indeed very blue. Cyanosis, we call it. Not enough oxygen in the blood. Peggy was only 17 years old and she had a throat infection which had caused tremendous swelling. The old timers called it quinsy. The docs now call it peritonsillar abscess. She had it around both tonsils. When she was admitted to the hospital earlier in the day, she was started on intravenous penicillin with the hope that total occlusion of the airway would not occur. But despite our treatment, the dreadful moment arrived. Peggy was unresponsive, her vital signs were fading and death was imminent. No time to go to surgery, so we exposed her neck and thrust a pillow under her shoulders. A quick alcohol prep to the area and the tracheotomy set was opened. She didn't need anesthesia. I took the knife and incised the skin over her trachea (windpipe). I quickly dissected through the muscles to the cartilaginous rings of the trachea. I thrust the knife into the windpipe and opened it up. The tracheotomy tube was inserted and the obstruction was relieved. Peggy sucked in a gasp of wonderful air and as she continued to breathe her blue color quickly turned to pink. That was a close call, too close. She began to move her hand and it came up to her neck and she felt the tracheotomy tube. She opened her eyes and looked at me and I told her what had happened. She understood but couldn't speak to me because of the tube in her throat. Peggy recovered and the penicillin did its work. The swelling subsided. She went home and later her tracheotomy tube was removed. The opening slowly closed by natural healing. She left the clinic after her final visit and I never saw her again.

Peggy was one of the thousands treated at our hospital in the hills of Troublesome Creek, Perry County, Kentucky. It was in the winter of 1956. Few doctors were available for people in those days and hospitals were few and far between. By today's standards, the practice of medicine and surgery was rather primitive and we worked more for love than for money. Many people were unemployed and many were impoverished. Coal miners were out of work because of mechanization and they were forced to leave their homes in order to find work in distant places.

After 20 years of working night and day, knee deep in disease and elbow deep in blood, the family needed a change, for living was difficult in this isolated area. We moved to the rolling hills of southern Indiana. After 17 years more of doctoring, I wrote my story and published my first book, *Refcrees, Docs And God* (Journal Of A Country Doctor). The Black

Gold Festival at Hazard, Kentucky was on. Many of my former friends and patients would still be in the area. I wanted to go back. When mountain folk like you, they love you, and they don't forget. I arranged for a booth at the festival and advertised my arrival in the local newspaper. For two days I was hugged and welcomed big time. I saw people I hadn't seen for years. We reminisced, told stories, and we had a ball. I sold books, 400 in all.

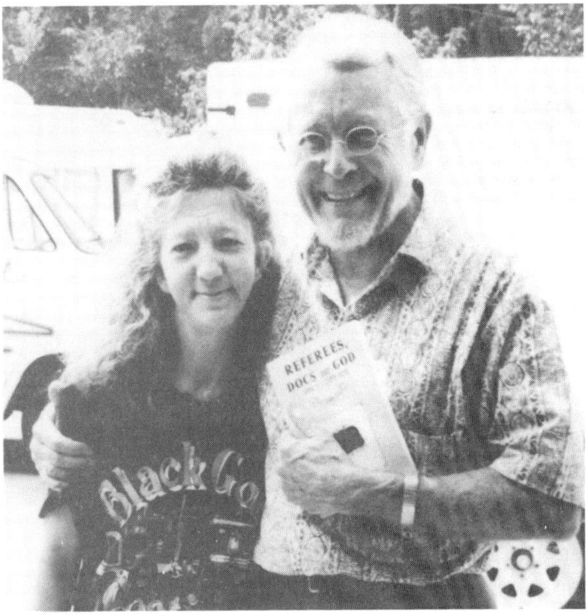

Black Gold Festival, Hazard, Kentucky, Summer 1990. Peggy and her doctor.

On the second afternoon, a middle-aged woman stood in front of my booth and looked at my display and at me. She was simply dressed and didn't seem to possess the courage to come up and speak to me. I got up and went out to her. She asked if I was really Dr. Martin. I nodded that I was. She looked at me and said, "You saved my life." She pulled her shirt down and exposed the scar on her neck. Immediately I knew who she was. It was Peggy. She said she wanted to come by and thank me even though she couldn't afford to buy my book. I reached for a copy, turned to page 21 and showed her where I had relayed the story of the lifesaving operation 51 years previously. I looked at her and she looked at me. We hugged each other. I gave her the book and she was gone.

That experience I will never forget. To me that is the bottom line of what doctoring is all about. I got something money couldn't buy. The stress of medical school and the practice of medicine is worth it when one can experience this kind of joy. It helps to compensate for the inevitable disappointments, frustrations, fatigue, and failures that await one as he faces the real world.

Johnny Gown In The Headlight

It was early fall at Homeplace clinic and hospital in my beloved Kentucky mountains. Mary arrived in early labor. Her man, John, brought her over in his pickup from up the holler where they lived with their 12 children. John's first woman had died and left him with the children. It didn't take him long to find another woman.

The labor started off badly and before it was over, it was a disaster. I ordered the usual demerol and scopolamine. That turned out to be a bad decision. Instead of obtaining relief, she became agitated, I mean really agitated, and she was big and strong. Our OB nurse was big too, but not strong enough. The patient knocked the nurse down and ran out of the back door of the hospital. By that time it was dark outside but that didn't stop Mary. Wearing nothing but her johnny gown she disappeared into the darkness. I was on call and the nurse put in a frantic call to me. Our house was only 50 yards from the hospital and I always slept in my scrub suit. When I heard the news I backed out my Ford, stopped at the hospital door and picked up the nurse. Down the road to the highway we went. Which way to go? Up or down the road? We made our decision and we drove slowly down the road looking for Mary. After a short drive around the first bend, we saw her johnny gown in the headlight and she was trying to go over the fence toward Troublesome Creek. We pulled up, got out and grabbed her! She fought a first-class struggle. We got her into the back seat of my two-door Ford and that was about the hardest job in the management of total labor. Back to the hospital we went and back to bed with great difficulty. She was still determined not to crawl back into that labor bed. It quickly became obvious that terminating the labor by the quickest means was our only hope. By this time Mary was wild. She had a full-blown acute psychosis and there was no way on earth we would let her deliver spontaneously. She would have dropped that baby in the hallway or in the parking lot or wherever. I called Dr. Keith Cameron, my associate. "Keith," I said, "We have to do a section." I explained the situation to him as he blinked his sleepy eyes in disbelief. With at least four people holding Mary on the stretcher, we took her to the OR fighting all the way. Restraints and OR straps were put in place. Pentathol was injected into the vein while holding her arm rigidly. She relaxed, went to sleep and the OR crew breathed a sigh of relief. After the prep, drape, and incision the baby was delivered in good shape.

A few days later, John showed up. It was pitiful to see him listen to the wild tale about his Mary. He looked at the ground the whole time. He wouldn't look me in the face. He was sober and ashamed. Finally, he said, "Doc, ole buddy, when I lost my woman I had twelve head of youngins to look after and I married quick, I had to."

Mary and baby and John disappeared down the hill in the pickup truck a few days later. I am not sure if I ever saw Mary again.

I wonder what ever happened to those 13 children. Blest are we who have had the good fortune to have capable and caring parents. Cursed are those who have not. As we sit in judgment on the sinner, the thief, the murderer, and the psychopath, we must remember that they may have been reared in a similar atmosphere. Those of us who have achieved some degree of success likely were blessed with a home that made that accomplishment possible.

Hazard, Perry County, Kentucky A City On Top Of The Mountains

Change is the name of the game in America. The changes in life and lifestyle in the past 50 years are mind boggling. We all know that. There is very little in life that has not undergone an unbelievable change. Oh, I know, there still is birth, death and taxes and yes, we still like to eat, like to love and like to fight. But beyond this, life "ain't the same, brother!" I have lived on the east coast, west coast, and in the midwest. I have lived in the hills and in the flat land. Change is everywhere; no area is untouched. I believe that Hazard, Kentucky demonstrates changes in a unique and amazing way. Thirty-six years ago I went to the area with my family. The roads coming in from every direction were narrow, winding and treacherous in the winter time. My children went to Williams Branch one-room school were Cora Combs taught all five grades. There were no telephones at home or in the hospital. We were out in the boonies — isolated. Flat or bottom land was at a premium and to find a place to build meant carving out a chunk of hillside to form a narrow shelf on which to build your house. The town of Hazard was over two mountains from our home. The business section of Hazard was strung out along the North Fork of the Kentucky River. Flooding was frequent and devastating. Houses were on the hillsides and often precariously perched and access was not all that easy. To grow and expand was virtually impossible.

All of this has undergone a profound change. I don't be lieve there is a place in the United States of America where changes could possibly be any more dramatic than Hazard,

Kentucky. Three and four-lane highways have now made access a spectacular pleasure instead of a dangerous enterprise. I used to take a jeep on a home medical call up Big Branch of Ball to Bearville. I was in and out of the creek for several miles and the trip was slow and rough. Now Bearville is on either side of a gorgeous four-lane highway which leads to Hindman, the county seat. The first time I drove to Bearville on this giant roller coaster road, I couldn't have been more excited if I had been in a rocket en route to the moon.

The city has now expanded to the mountain tops. The strip mines have leveled a number of mountain tops, making it possible to build a regional hospital of 160 beds, shopping center, and motels. Valleys have been filled in as hillsides have been carved out and more flat land is available for commercial use. A community college has expanded with remarkable success and has over 1,800 students. Restaurants and fast foods of every description are to be found. The doctors and dentists have a new office building alongside the hospital. A hundred bed psychiatric hospital is being built. Coal is still mined but fewer men are employed due to mechanization. Tourism is becoming an important part of the economic life of the area. Leaders of the community often have been people of wealth and influence and have been respected because of their dedication to the idea of making Hazard and Perry County a better place to live. They are to be congratulated for a job unusually well done. Hazard has won numerous awards in Kentucky for its outstanding progress. Hazard has gone to the mountain top for sure!

Williams Branch

Williams Branch — oh Williams Branch — how many are the memories I have of thee! Homeplace Community Center, my home of 20 years, is located at the mouth of the stream where it entered Troublesome Creek. The road up the branch was dirt and rock, full of holes, and virtually impassible difficult as it is to practice medicine night and day for decades, it is always better to be the doctor than the patient. I recall when Dr. Williams came to Hazard in the early 1950's and took the place of our recently deceased internist, Martin Palmer, M.D. Williams soon established himself as a competent practitioner with excellent diagnostic skills. He pushed and shoved to raise the standards of medical care in the Hazard area. In the early 1960's he took advanced training in a special hospital unit. Subsequently, he initiated the first coronary care unit in the Hazard Appalachian Regional Hospital. He was meticulous in his medical examinations and wrote letters second to none to his referring doctors. They were outstanding in their clarity and straight to the point. Seldom did he err in his diagnosis and judgment.

My children and his children have been close friends through the years and this has kept us in touch. Along with my other medical colleagues in Hazard, I say goodbye to a friend and fellow practitioner and offer this tribute to his family, friends, and patients.

Dog Surgery

I should have known better but I didn't. I do now. When I first went to Homeplace Hospital I was not too busy during the early building phase of the practice so I was hot to take on about anything. I did and sometimes to my regret. One such regretful incidence was as follows:

One of our staff nurses got a new female dog. The nurse wanted it spayed so she asked me to do it if I was able and willing. I was eager to do it. I didn't know much about dog surgery or dog anatomy but I didn't think that would matter. I did know that to spay a dog you had to surgically remove the ovaries and so, on the appointed day, we put the dog to sleep and I made the incision in the pelvic area, as I would for a human. I found the uterus and the tubes quite well but I couldn't find the ovaries. I finally discovered that they were way up out of the pelvis, quite unaccessible to my pelvic incision. I had to extend the incision upward a considerable distance in order to gain exposure enough to remove the ovaries. I finally managed to get the procedure done. We took the dog to the hospital basement where she spent the night. She was not at all happy. She was up all night whining and howling and bouncing around and generally making herself a nuisance and I am sure she was quite miserable too. She kept some of the patients awake which was not appreciated. It was my first and last spay job I can assure you.

Lesson: 1. I recommend that doctors stick with people and Veterinarians take care of the dogs; 2. Overconfidence can sometimes get us into trouble; 3. Be sure of your limitations before starting a new procedure; 4. Tread on familiar ground if possible. Anyhow the dog didn't get pregnant so I guess I did the right thing.

Glimpses Of Homeplace

Bad Headache

I had a fascinating 20 years practicing in rural Appalachia. One of the reasons was my relationship with the country people from up the hollers. I think I can safely say that I loved them and they loved me. It is as simple as that. They were not very compliant, they were prone to put things off till disease was in full bloom, and they lived a sort of disorganized life from my point of view. Nevertheless, I really enjoyed being their doctor. One reason was the way that they expressed themselves. The mountain man described his illness in a way unique to the mountains. He painted you a word picture. Early on in my experience a man came in to see me and he told me about his headaches. "Doc, ole buddy, this headache has been follering me for yars. I can't shun it!" "Doc, sometimes it feels just like you would put a 45 caliber pistol between my eyeballs and pull the trigger." I got the message.

Full Stomach

A man came in to see me one day because of "high blood." He meant hypertension. He was fat, real fat, and he always had garlic on his breath. Said he, "garlic is good for high blood, doc." It was so bad I could hardly go into the room and stay longer than a minute or two. In my youth as a doctor, I thought that preaching to the patients about bad health habits could make a difference. Frankly, experience has taught me after 45 years that preaching seldom works. Anyhow, I always managed to get him weighed each visit and fuss about his weight problem. He didn't change, of course. Finally one day he said, "Doc, honey, you might as well stop talking about my fat stomach. When I die, I will die with a full stomach, and that is all there is to it." The men frequently used the friendly word, "honey" when talking to each other. So I said I would stop it, because it wasn't doing any good anyhow. I never saw him again. He did die, suddenly, a week or so later and I suspect with a full stomach.

Christmas Firecracker

It was customary in the Kentucky hills for the boys and playful men to shoot off firecrackers at Christmastime. Where I came from it was always reserved for the 4th of July. Well, anyway, firecrackers are dangerous as we all know and some of us have found out by experience. One Christmas I had seven firecracker injuries in a row from Christmas Eve until Christmas night. The injuries resulted in hand and face wounds and some were real bad. The daring boys played a game called *chicken*. Two boys would light the fuse of a cannon cracker and see who would hold it the longest before he tossed it out of danger range. Once in a while, a brave but foolish guy would exceed the limit and would have the thing explode in his hand. Fingers were badly bruised and sometimes permanently damaged by the loss of tissue. Mainly, fingernails and finger tips. The last injury that year was tragic. A young brave man engaged in this daring sport with a buddy and he was not the chicken. He held it the longest but too late. As he attempted at the last minute to pitch it to safety, the cannon cracker exploded near his face and badly damaged his right eye. He ended up with significant permanent damage to that eye. His left eye was already blind from a previous injury. For one foolish moment, he was reduced to a state of disabling dependence for life.

D-Con Club

Thirty years ago the treatment of acute myocardial infarction (heart attack) was vastly different from today. It was diagnosed by a clinical impression and EKG. There were no enzymes to help, no echocardiogram, no stress test, no catheterization, no angioplasty, no open heart surgery — only bed rest, and morphine for pain. An oxygen tent was available as necessary and digitalis and quinidine for rhythm disturbances. Mercuhydrin was available by injection for congestive heart failure and fluid collection. We put all of our patients with a heart attack on anti-coagulant drugs to prevent complications. First we used a drug called dicumerol but it was hard to manage and there were often bleeding complications. Hedulin, a new drug, became available and it was easier to manage. Then, coumadin was available and we still use that to this very day. You may or may not know that warfarin which is the generic name for coumadin, is also the ingredient in rat poison. Rats eat warfarin to an excess and bleed to death internally and so we get rid of rats and mice. We give small controlled doses of warfarin to humans to slow up blood clotting and, in this way, save lives and extend the length of life for those who have been stricken with a myocardial infarction. Frankly, I was impressed with the effectiveness of this program. Now we limit its use only to certain people. On Fridays at Homeplace we had what we called D-Con Club Day. This consisted of people who had had a heart attack and were coming back to check their clotting time in order that we might properly dose them with coumadin. It turned out to be a real winner. They became a support group for one another and the quality of life I am sure was improved because these people met together and joked together and helped one another. As they told stories and jokes it helped them endure the uncertainty of the future and made life a bit more tolerable. Some of those patients are likely alive even to this day because of "rat poison."

Breck Holliday

Breck was and still is a great guy in my book. He was general fix-it man at Homeplace. If it was broken, Breck usually could fix it. He did farm work, yard work, maintenance at the hospital, plumbing, electrical work, and was telephone line repairman. One night we were doing a caesarean section in the operating room and a storm was raging with lightning and thunder and torrents of rain. The emergency generator came on when the electric current went out all of a sudden. However, the light in the operating room was not that good with our generator and we really needed the current restored as soon as possible. We called Breck. He came at once, put on his rain gear and took what I thought was a great risk to himself. He had a wooden pole, real long with a tool at one end that he used to make some corrections in the big transformer on the utility pole outside the hospital. I was watching him from the window. It was dark. It was raining like cats and dogs. As he worked, at times the sparks would fly in the vicinity of the working area at the end of the pole. Finally, the lights came on as he restored contact by fixing the blown fuse. I wondered if he would live through that experience. A brave man he was, a good man. We finished the operation and mom and babe were doing well.

Biting Kind

One winter night a patient came into our emergency room at Homeplace Clinic with an injury to his ear. It was bleeding and deformed. We got lots of emergencies because our clinic and hospital, although small, was open for business 24 hours a day, seven days a week, 365 days a year, and one doctor was always there, either in the hospital or 50 yards away at his house. So we were busy. Patients knew that they would get prompt attention.

Anyhow, I examined the ear. The patient was a bit drunk and he smelled of booze. But he cooperated and let me do my thing. Part of his ear simply was gone, torn away as it were. I was curious and asked the usual questions. Whereupon, he responded as best he could with slurred speech, "It was plumb bitten off, doc." I did as good a plastic job as I could and sent him out.

A few nights later about one in the morning, a patient presented himself to the emergency room and the nurse called me. This guy had a nose injury and was bleeding. I slept in my scrubs, which made it easier to get up and down through the night. I got out of bed, put my shoes on and went the 50 yards to the hospital emergency room. I examined this patient and he too was a bit drunk and I came to find out that he had a portion of his nose bitten off during a fight. It was in the same tavern as the previous case. My curiosity was increasing about these two situations. I did the best I could to patch him. No doubt he returned to get even with his assailant. The saga continued and a few nights later a third victim of biting during a tavern brawl came into our emergency room. It was the same tavern, different patient. This you won't believe but, so help me, it's true. This guy was a bit drunk and he complained about an injury to his tongue. I asked him to stick the tongue out which he did, and low and behold, the tip of his tongue was missing. He said it was bitten off in a fight. Upon further questioning it seems to me that his assailant was the same man involved in both the cases I had recently seen. I asked him what kind of a guy this man was. He apparently had bitten three people, an ear, a nose, and finally a tongue. "Doc," he said, "he was the bitin' kind!" End of story.

Baby Blank

We had our share of premature babies at Homeplace. We did not have the luxury of a neonatal intensive care nursery as is now available in medical centers. No pediatrician, no neonatologist, no way to intubate and give intravenous feedings to tiny babies too young to survive on their own. And so some babies that we lost no doubt could be saved today with modern technology. We did have the Armstrong Incubator and later we obtained the Isolette, which was the cadillac of incubators for our preemies. One day a Mrs. Blank came to our hospital in labor but she was much too early, about seven months along as I recall. She proceeded to deliver a delicate tiny female, preemie, which of course, we called Baby Blank. She survived the ordeal of delivery and the weeks of special preemie care that was necessary. Ultimately, she went home with mamma and pappa Blank and I presumed lived happily ever after. In Hazard at the 1990 Black Gold Festival, some 25 years later, I was greeting friends and former patients and selling my book, *Referees, Docs And God (Journal Of A Country Doctor)*. A smiling man came up on one occasion and introduced himself as "Mr. Blank." Wow! The wheels turned but I couldn't get it straight for a moment who he was. Then he said, "You remember Baby Blank, don't you?" Whereupon, it all came back to me and with intense joy I heard him describe Baby Blank at the present. A healthy and successful adult doing her thing and making her way in the world. All of our long days and nights of hard work with that tiny premature baby paid off.

Cat Bite Hysteria

Time: about 1960. Place: Buckhorn Children's Home on Buckhorn Creek in Breathitt County on the North Fork of the

Kentucky River. Persons: about 30 children and the house parents. A stray cat appeared on the scene and many of the children were delighted to have a new orphan come into their midst. Over the next few days they petted the cat and some were scratched. Finally, two or three were bitten and at this point measures were taken to corral the friendly but turned vicious feline. The cat was isolated with the intention of disposing of it one way or another the next day. The next day came but the cat, alas, was found dead. Someone suspected that maybe, just maybe, the cat might have died of rabies. The head was sent to the State Health Department laboratory and sure enough, the dreaded answer came back that indeed the cat had died of rabies. Now that disease can be fatal to humans as well and all those children who played with the cat were believed to be candidates for immunization, especially those who had been bitten or scratched. Homeplace Clinic was selected to do the job immunizing these children. Memory fails to tell how many kids were inoculated in the shot series but there was a bunch. I suspect most if not all of the 30 kids in the Children's Home were given 21 shots each in a series to prevent rabies. We generally gave the vaccine in the fat layer of the abdomen just beneath the skin. You could imagine the job on our hands of giving 21 shots to 30 kids. Many of these children didn't understand what was happening and were terrified. Some were quite young and others were older but all were apprehensive and getting 21 shots in the abdomen was a nerve-racking experience for all concerned. We lived through it and no one got rabies. I doubt if there are many cat lovers out there who once lived at Buckhorn Children's Home.

Big Tall Pine

In my first year at Homeplace I was cutting the grass one day and ran over a little pine tree that was on the hillside. It was about two feet tall. I didn't amputate it, I just knocked it over and partly uprooted it. I hated that. I had recently lost a beautiful fir tree I had purchased from the nursery which

I had planted out in front of our house. So I thought I had nothing to lose by planting that poor little assaulted pine in the bare spot. I took three or four whacks with the mattock and made a hole in the hard clay ground, stuck in the pine, covered the roots, gave it a shot of water, and forgot about it. No problem and it grew. I went back to Homeplace 18 years later, 35 years since the tree was planted. It was huge! Twice as tall as my house, shedding its needles on the roof and all over the place. This points out a fact of life. The pedigree species sometimes fail where the ordinary flourishes. Maybe that is the way it is in life too, you reckon?

Pink Lady's Slipper

People used to bring me gifts at Homeplace through the years: garden stuff aplenty, sometimes pickled eggs, pickled corn, and shucky beans. Eulah Mae Holliday knew that I loved wild flowers and often went on wild flower pilgrimages in the Smoky Mountains. She also knew that I was successful in transplanting some species on a shaded hillside in back of my house. I had found some yellow lady's slippers but never any pink ones. One day she brought me two pink lady's slippers, wonderful! I planted them and watched over them like a mother hen. They flourished. Each spring they bloomed and I was there to enjoy their delicacy. One spring as I was entering my arboretum, I saw a rabbit nibbling away at my lady's slippers and that sucker cut off both stems and the lovely and delicate lady's slipper blossoms lay on the ground. I almost cried. And they didn't live happily ever after. Matter of fact, they never bloomed again all through the years that I was at Homeplace.

A few years after I left Homeplace I went back for a visit. I saw old friends who still worked at the clinic and toured the grounds. I went by my house and just looked around and reminisced. Then I walked out into the back yard and onto the hillside arboretum where my wild flowers were. I wondered if they were still blooming. It was spring time and so the time was right. There were the yellow lady's slippers, the red phlox, the wild iris, the jack in the pulpit, the trillium, and the wild geranium. There was the blood root and the hepatica. I went on further and looked to see if the pink lady's slippers were still coming up. To my amazement, they were not only up but blooming once more after all these years of nothing. Lesson — don't give up too quick.

Parnate

One patient of mine at Homeplace Clinic through the years was the wife of a clergyman, one of the "outsiders," and the term that was used to characterize these people was that of a Christian worker. They performed religious duties, social work undertakings, and generally were jacks of all trades in trying to help people. She was afflicted with the monster called depression, and had been off and on much of her life. In the 1950's we had no antidepressant medications whatsoever. To cope with this malady, some became drug abusers, particularly with alcohol. Some committed suicide and others to whom expense was not an issue, took months or years in counseling and psychotherapy. With her, no treatment was able to deal with the problem. She suffered a lot and so did her family and friends.

About this time the first of the antidepressants came onto the medical scene. It was called Parnate. It is known as an MAO inhibitor drug which enables some people to function better emotionally. Before long, she came in for a check up. We put her on Parnate and gave her the diet adjustment necessary for those on this kind of drug. She took it for three to four weeks. She got better. In about six weeks there was a noticeable improvement in her functioning and she was feeling better. She was less depressed, and virtually functioning as she once had as a wife and mother. This is not to say that she remained a well person because she had her ups and downs but overall her life was much more productive and pleasant while she remained on this drug.

Since Parnate came out, many other chemicals have appeared on the scene and because of this, countless lives have been saved and many people are able to function normally or almost normally instead of living in the gravel pit of despair. Antidepressant medications must be taken by some people daily indefinitely just like a diabetic requires insulin to live. Unfortunately, depression is not an "okay" disease. There is still the feeling out there that one should be able to rise above this disease unassisted. That is just as wrong as it would be to say that one should be able to overcome diabetes by simply deciding to do so and to live above it and to deny it. Diabetes is inherited and requires insulin in many cases. Depression, likewise, runs in families and requires daily medication in many instances.

Rusty Water

The Martins arrived at Homeplace in 1954 and set up housekeeping with their three children. Among numerous other duties in our house was the matter of weekly washing of clothes and other items. We had a spin dry washer. In one tub the washing took place and in the other tank the washed clothes were spun dry by centrifugal force. We were warned that the well water at Homeplace was rusty and smelled like slightly aged eggs. Not until the first wash was completed did we realize just how rusty the water really was. The clean clothes looked absolutely brown from the filtered out rust in the water. The sheets were a mess, the skirts, underwear, everything a mess. Whereupon the lady of the house exclaimed that if the water situation was not corrected, she had done her last washing at Homeplace.

I got out the Yellow Pages of the phone directory — no I didn't, we didn't have any telephone at Homeplace. So I made inquiries in the town of Hazard, our county seat, about our dilemma. I found that the Culligan Water Filter Service People were available. I contacted them and they came out to our house and installed a system of filters which removed the rust and much of the sulfur compounds from the water. It worked, it worked, it worked! Because of Culligan, I reckon, I could safely say that the Martins stayed for 20 years in the mountains. Sometimes, little things, make a big difference.

Bad Foot

One day at the clinic a young man came in using crutches in order to walk. His right foot he held up and couldn't walk on it. The nurse then brought him into the examination room, took his history, vital signs, and removed his shoe and looked at his foot. She saw an unbelievable sight. I was informed to be prepared for a shock. I entered his room, talked to the man and then examined his foot. The bottom of his foot was covered by what we doctors call plantar warts. The entire walking surface of his foot was covered by warts of all sizes. I counted 100 warts and just quit counting. I was only half way through. I wasn't sure what to do. In those days we used 40 percent salicylic acid plaster as we do today and started his treatment. I saw him on a few occasions and was beginning to see some improvement. I saw him for the last time before I left the mountains and came to Salem. At this point he was still walking on crutches and had a long long way to go. I have often wondered whatever happened to that boy. Did he ever get rid of the warts? Those of you who have had one or two plantar warts or perhaps as many as ten know just what trouble they can cause with walking. I treated one patient for almost a year to get rid of 10 or 15 warts on her foot; can you imagine how long it would take to get rid of 200?

Broken Arm x Two

A kid fell off his bike and got a nasty fracture of both bones of his right forearm, the radius and the ulna. There was marked angulation (the arm was crooked). I mean real crooked. We put him to sleep and reduced the fracture (bent it back to straighten it). We got a good reduction and the arm was straight. A long arm cast was applied from the upper arm to his hand which is standard procedure. I told him the break would require longer than usual to heal being in that location and he would have to keep his cast on 10-12 weeks at least. At the end of six or seven weeks he wanted it off. He begged me. I said, "No!" The boy persuaded his mom to request that I remove it and she backed him up and wanted it off regardless of my advice. So off it came and I warned him again about falling and hurting that arm. He and his mother left. I went on working and saw a few more patients when low and behold who should come back hurting and crying with a bent and crooked arm just like he had first experienced. Yes, my patient had gone out of the clinic and jumped out of the car and ran down the bank to the creek. He slipped and fell and the fracture occurred just like I had warned him only this time it was worse. Another anesthetic, and another reduction, and another cast. Another seven weeks, no 14 weeks, and he learned a lesson and so did I.

First Glimpse And Last Look At Homeplace

It was in the spring of 1954 that I drove with my dad to Ary, Kentucky, deep in the heart of the Kentucky mountains to visit Homeplace. I came to talk with Dr. Keith Cameron, MB. CHB. Dr. Cameron was an Englishman having been born and reared in Liverpool, England, and having gone to the university there to study medicine. He had gone to China as a medical missionary where he had remained for a number of years until the Communists took over the country and he had to leave. He had married an American lady while in China and instead of going to England he came to the States and eventually to Homeplace Hospital. It was the sort of work he had always wanted to do. He worked out in the bush so to speak and he needed help. He was alone. I needed Homeplace. I don't know for sure who needed whom most. It doesn't matter. I wanted to go overseas and be another *Burma surgeon* or another Albert Schweitzer but the monster of depression reared its ugly head and struck me a blow. That shattered temporarily my confidence but after my recovery I wondered what I would do. I was hesitant to go overseas at this point. I had to prove myself first. And the opportunity came to do a job not overseas, but in my home state of Kentucky in the mountains. The area was medically deprived and I wanted and needed to be needed. And so to Homeplace I went. I found a beautiful valley with a number of buildings and in the midst the hospital and clinic built of native stone, and a lovely site it was. I found a man there, Dr. Cameron, 10 years older than myself, whom I instantly liked and he liked me. Dad and I drove the winding mountain road back to the Bluegrass and on to Louisville where I was finishing my surgical residency. I had found my place but when time came to go I got scared. I knew that after being at Homeplace a month or so, Dr. Cameron had asked for a three-week vacation and I would be alone. Clinic and hospital, on call 24-hours-a-day, seven-days a week, and I would be seeing patients and doing everything that had to be done. I would have to be family doctor, obstetrician, gynecologist, surgeon, pediatrician, psychiatrist, dermatologist, cardiologist, orthopedist, emergency room physician, I had to be it all. All of this for $500.00 a month and a house for my family. There were no extras, no package deals. But I had agreed to go and I couldn't back down. I went, I survived, I even eventually flourished and I loved the people and they loved me. For 20 years I did my thing and then one day I had my last glimpse of Homeplace. Keith and I went up on the hill overlooking Homeplace to get a picture of us together with the lovely Homeplace Valley in its idyllic setting in the background. My son, Donnie, went along and took my Rollei Reflex Camera to make the picture. It was a good one. It shows two doctors sitting and talking on the hill overlooking the setting where for 20 years they worked together. We looked at the place where we worked side by side through thick and thin. Where babies were born, where people died, where pain was relieved, and where pain was inflicted on the doctor

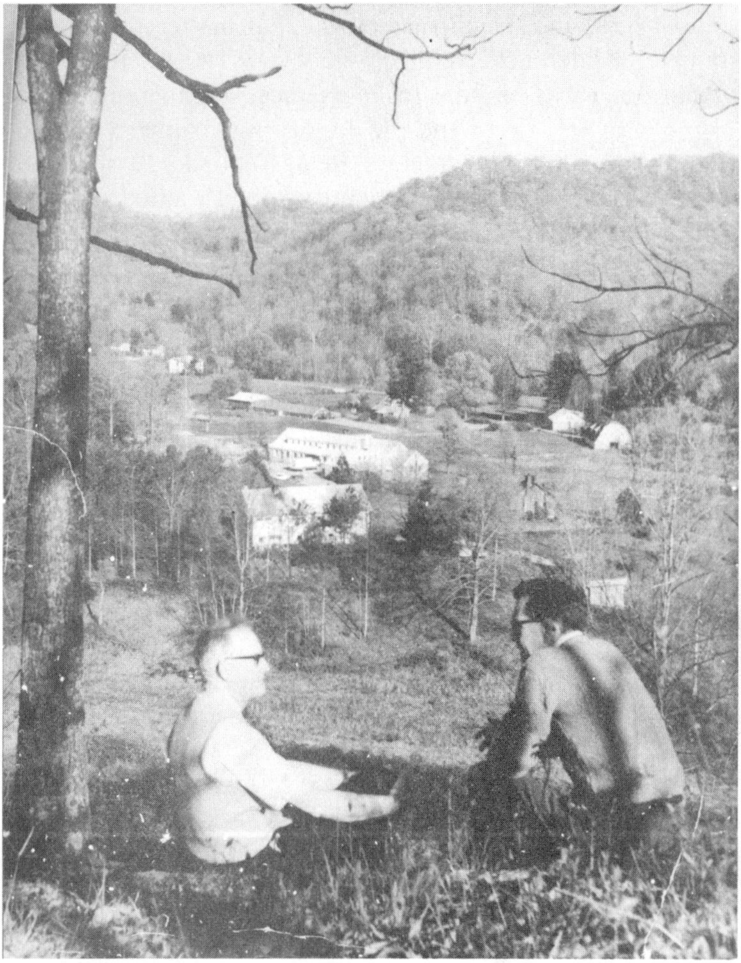

Homeplace Community Center, Spring, 1969. Clinic and hospital center building. Keith Cameron, MB.CHB., (left) and Donald L. Martin, MD, in foreground.

when he felt he had messed up a case. We never had an argument. We were different in many ways but we had no conflict. He was a true gentleman, honorable, dedicated, and a role model for me. We had similar priorities and similar goals, and that made our working together possible. The last glimpse, a parting look, and we said goodbye.

I go back at least once a year to make my pilgrimage to Homeplace. I see some of the same staff members working and it is just a wonderful experience to go back but it is not the same. It can't be. Time marches on. On one occasion a mountain woman embraced me and said, "Doc Martin, why don't you come back and stay?" I responded, "You have plenty of doctors now and you don't need me anymore." And then she said, "but, doc honey, they will never be another doctor like you." I am sure that is not true but that is the way she felt. I need that. I always did and I guess I always will and I can't apologize that I'm needy.

Trip To Yesterday

Mid-September 1990 found me in the land I left almost 17 years ago and seeing people I served and loved. Ah, yes, I was in Hazard, Perry County Kentucky, in the heart of the coal fields for the Black Gold Festival. I had heard that it was big time and it was! I mean great big time. Crowds so big you could move only with caution. Entertainment, old home week, buying and selling crafts, and what not. Food, fun and parades. Wow! I loved it. I advertised my coming by newspaper and word of mouth. I obtained a booth among the other exhibitors and sellers in order to meet my old friends and patients. I sold 400 copies of my book, *Referees, Docs And God.* I wouldn't have missed it for the world. I saw folk I hadn't seen in 30 years.

I spent two and a half days at the festival. A pretty girl came up to me and informed me that the leading story in my book was about her mother's sister. Amazing! She was the young mother dying from blood loss following a delivery complicated by DIC Syndrome. Fibrinogen was flown in from the University of Louisville Medical School and saved her life.

Others came by and identified themselves. A number of people in their 20's and 30's shook my hand or hugged me saying that I was the doctor who had delivered them at Homeplace Hospital. What a joy and what delight! A man came up and said, "Doc, you remember my dog? I brought him to the clinic and asked you if you'd sew up his cut leg. You said you would provided I snuck him in the back door and departed the same way. You didn't want me to take him out there through the waiting room which was full of people waiting to see you. Doc, I will never forget you."

The mayor and his wife came by and other important people did, too. All sorts of folk came by. It was an experience that I shall never again have and I shall treasure it to my grave. To me this is the bottom line of what life is all about. Oh, I know that I have an advantage in as much as I enjoy relating to others. So many do not do this with ease or joy. I consider myself to be blessed and indeed fortunate to have the capacity to enter into these kinds of experiences. I believe I learned a lot from the mountain people about this sort of thing. Mountain folk are people-oriented. So many do not have an abundance of things to get in their way and so people have become important. I like that. This is where it is, I do believe.

And so at Black Gold Days the folk came from near and far and they came from the hollers, they came from the towns, and they came from wherever. Many are unable to get to the big cities, and so these local festivals give them an opportunity to visit, swap tales, spend some money, but mainly to do somcthing different and be identified with the crowd. At festival time, barriers are broken down. The mayor and the garbage man walk side by side. There are no rich or poor, black or white, smart or dumb, all are simply festival folk doing their thing. It's great. It's American. It's fun.

I do so very much appreciate the response of my friends and patients who took time to come by and greet me, many with a hug, all with a handshake and smile. That helps so much in a world of pain and suffering, disappointment, sweat and grief. I hope to be a part of Black Gold again before I check out and become a memory.

Tidbits For Young Doctors

1. Some say doctors have it made and get more than they deserve. This is true in some cases. I got more than I deserved doctoring the sick and suffering. I got tuberculosis, hepatitis B, three law suits and stress induced recurrent depression.

2. To be shipshape at times demands conformity to the shape of the ship. If we keep bottling it up, eventually there will be an explosion.

3. Women tend to complain and men are stubborn.

4. Sensitivity to the needs of others is a great asset to the counselor. On the other hand, it does exact its toll and after a day one is drained.

5. Working nights in the emergency room at Louisville General Hospital for two years, as a student, let me know what being a doctor was all about. I saw it all, did it all, and felt confident to face it all, come what may, tomorrow.

6. Studying about germs and disease was one thing; seeing it in action in the patient was another. Experiencing it yourself and being the patient is altogether different.

7. It takes twelve years of school to become a doctor and the price is high. In the learning process we are only on first base. We may be smart at graduation day but we won't be wise until we have experienced the medical battle-field, where bullets fly and blood flows and where some live and some die.

8. Help me, oh Lord, not to spend effort, time, and money on that which cannot and should not be fixed, but help me to do my best to fix that which can be, and give me the wisdom to know the difference.

9. Help me, oh Lord, to fly when I should fly, crawl when I should crawl, and give me the wisdom to know when to do what.

10. You are blessed if you don't have incapacitating mood swings. Be cautious in your judgment of those who do, it may be beyond their control.

11. The war on cancer is being slowly won but the war on drugs is not going well.

12. Try to be pleasant. That helps at the sick bed.

13. Keep up to date magazines in each examination room. Your patients will wait more patiently for you.

14. Sometimes we feel the sting of ingratitude as we deal with suffering people but occasionally the "widow gives us her mite" as the person on food stamps brings us a fruit basket at Christmastime.

15. Doctors can diagnose many conditions simply by listening to the patient, but doing an examination will tell more and is impressive to the patient.

16. Don't play God. You are not that good.

17. Make a decision. Better to swing and miss than to be counted out on strikes.

18. Take the bull by the horns before you get gored.

19. It's not much fun to wait, but remember, a lot of people will wait on you.

20. It used to be doctor and patient relationships. Now it is doctor-patient-Medicare-Medicaid-third parties-peer review-joint commission-quality assurance-lawyers and next year there will be more.

21. It is bad enough to be sick but to have to pay to get well is worse.

22. Medical, surgical, and hospital bills are high. They better be good.

23. *Referees, Docs And God* must not make a mistake.

24. "But Doc, why do I get so fat? I don't eat a thing."

25. "But Doc, don't you think I have a lot of water in my body?"

26. Please don't stop smoking. My business would be cut in half!

27. If we took as much care of our stomachs as we do our gas tank, we would all be better off. If we treated our cars the same as we do our bodies, many of our autos would be disabled.

28 Hemorrhoids are no fun but a colostomy is worse.

29. The agitation of nicotine withdrawal is hell, but living with cancer is worse.

30. Chronic bronchitis is bad but end stage emphysema is hell.

31. Practicing medicine in America in the 1990's is frustrating and scary, but doctors and patients still come to America to be a part of the medical scene.

32. Hurry up and operate, the patient might get well.

33. Don't be surprised if the patient trusts the neighbor's advice more than yours.

34. Listen to the patient. If you listen long enough, you will be told the diagnosis.

35. Regardless of the blood alcohol level, the patient has "only had two beers."

36. Some patients don't pay their bills because their cigarette and booze bills are so high.

37. Some patients don't pay their bills because they are overcharged.

38. Some patients don't pay their bills because good intentions don't balance the account.

39. When the spouse accompanies the husband to the office and is in the room with him, you know why. He has been coerced or threatened and she wants to hear it straight from the doctor.

40. Kids will love you if you don't give shots.

41. Kids love you outside the office.

42. You will be called on to give curbstone consultations so be prepared.

43. Don't be an alarmist. It's easier to start a fire than to put one out.

44. Reassurance is the best thing you can prescribe in the office. Freely use it.

45. Take some chances for the good of humanity. You will not regret it.

46. When we are well and happy, we live as if there is no death. When we have had the sentence of death placed upon us by the medical realities, some of us die right then.

47. Blessed are you if you can lie down and go to sleep quickly and wake up refreshed.

48. Blessed are you if you have not been attacked by a legal buzzard circling constantly over the medical battlefield awaiting a carcass that can be devoured.

49. Burdens are tough to bear during the day but at night we bear them alone.

50. Tell the patient what you are going to do. Surprises in the doctor's office are for the birds.

51. Wash your hands.

52. Clean your glasses.

53. Clip and clean your nails.

54. Be neat.

55. Hindsight is 20/20 vision.

56. Foresight needs an expert.

57. A medical officer aboard a navy ship with a thousand healthy men is not paid for what he does, but he is paid to be available.

58. To be able to adjust to the new, and accept the inevitable is a great thing, and not every doctor can do this.

59. To be willing to treat the unworthy, the difficult, and the unlovely patient, is likewise a great thing; not every doctor will do this.

60. Massage your patient's back, not his pocketbook.

61. Pay attention to complaints of constipation. It may not be so important to you, but surely it is to your patient, especially the senior citizens.

62. When you have completed the examination of a patient and it is time to give your report to the family, be sure all appropriate and interested members are together, or else you will be repeating yourself. Second hand information is generally not as reliable as first hand.

63. Patients increasingly inform themselves about medical matters in order to assure themselves of better medical care. I doubt if that really helps. Doctors who "know the most" usually make the worst patients and complicate the medical decision making.

64. If you believe that a certain medicine will help your ailment, you are already on first base. If you believe it will not help you, you are likely to strike out.

65. Most of the cures of illness and healings from injury occur without the assistance of the doctor or the surgeon. This is not to suggest allowing nature to heal acute appendicitis, however. God and the surgeon work together.

66. Depression is: cloudy skies, prison walls, failure, rejection, hopelessness, terminal illness, it might have been, it will never be the same, sitting beside one's dying child, saying farewell to one you have loved.

67. Ecstasy is: a way of escape, love given in return, plans for tomorrow, recognition, a job well done, receiving a letter of thanks, found not guilty, emerging from deep depression.

68. Satisfaction is: feeling good about your life, having someone to love, being loved by someone, feeding a hungry person, saving a life, relieving pain, going to bed tired and getting up rested, helping someone and seeing them succeed.

69. The price you pay to be different can be great. Joseph Lister, father of modern surgical sterility, was laughed out of town for years. If you think you are right, stick to your guns.

Part Two:

Medical Stories And Health Care Issues

—1—
Amish Baby Buggy

My phone rang at 6:30 after a usual busy day at the office and an urgent request for my presence was made by the operating room nurse at Washington County Hospital. A familiar life-threatening scenario was unfolding. An Amish mother was in early labor at the hospital (with a prolapsed umbilical cord). This event happened at the clinic where an Amish midwife delivers many of her own people. The midwife knew that this would mean death of the baby unless quick intervention took place and rushed the mother to the hospital. The baby was alive but in grave danger of dying from deprivation of blood supply because of the prolapsed umbilical cord. With each labor pain, the baby's head would be pushed down against the umbilical cord which had managed to prolapse into the vagina to the outside world when the bag of water ruptured. This is a very unusual event but, on occasion, does occur. The patient was taken to surgery at once, but the surgeon was forty-five minutes away. Time was critical. I had done only one caesarean section in the past twenty years and that was under similar circumstances eight years ago. The mother was prepared for surgery as a team member pushed the baby's head up away from the cord and held it in that position until surgery could be accomplished. I quickly scrubbed and got into my gown and gloves. I rehearsed the steps of a low transverse uterine incision caesarean section as I scrubbed. My first fifteen years of practice in the Kentucky mountains saw me doing caesarean sections whenever they were required but that had been a long time ago.

The mother was put to sleep and the operation started. We couldn't empty the bladder with a catheter because of the doctor's fist in the vagina, holding the baby's head up away from the cord, attempting to save the baby's life. Care had to be taken not to damage the full bladder during the operation. Despite this disadvantage, the operation proceeded, the lower uterine segment of the uterus was entered and the baby was delivered. It was limp, blue, and gave no effort to breathe whatsoever. Meconium stained amniotic fluid gave evidence of the baby's precarious state. The cord was clamped and resuscitation began at once on the baby. The operation was completed and the mother was all right. The baby was intubated and the lungs were inflated. The blue color was replaced by pink as things improved. Finally, the baby began to move and it appeared it might survive. The helicopter (which we call the baby chopper) was summoned and it arrived with a special team to take care of the problem. After an hour or more of preparation work on the baby it was flown to Children's Hospital in Louisville.

Two days later I visited the baby in the neonatal nursery at Children's Hospital. It was the first time I had been in the hospital since its occupancy. I had observed it on a tour a few weeks before it had opened. As I walked into this massive room filled with newborns in various stages of illness in the neonatal period, I was utterly amazed with what I saw. It was like a beehive of activity with skilled personnel attending these newborns, all of which were critically ill and hooked up to ventilators, monitors, oxygen, tubes, and various means of life support. Because of the advancement of medical science, many will be alive tomorrow — because of the expertise practiced in that room. I introduced myself and was taken over to the baby that I had seen (in critical condition) two days previously. On this occasion the baby was relatively vigorous, it was off the ventilator and oral feedings were started. It was clear by this time that the baby had a good chance of survival. Forty-five years before, as a junior medical student in the old Children's Hospital, such a scene as this would have been impossible. Very little of the equipment that I saw in operation that day was in existence then. The advancement in care and technique was awesome to think about. When I considered that this was an Amish baby, coming from a culture so vastly different from our own, the striking differences were even more obvious. This baby, if it survived, would grow up with horses and buggies, black dresses and bonnets, no electricity, no telephone, only the simple life. It lived because of all that modern science and medical advances had brought about, a staggering thought for sure.

A few weeks passed and I was eager to hear about the baby. I was able to get word to the family by contacting the midwife who had attended the mother. A short while later, when I arrived at the office, my nurse informed me that the Amish father of the baby I had delivered had left me a present and he had already disappeared in his buggy. I went downstairs to my private office and there I saw perhaps the most beautiful and unique piece of furniture I had ever seen. An Amish rocker, hand-made of oak and another beautiful wood that I did not recognize. Only exceeding its beauty and uniqueness was its comfort. It fit perfectly, it rocked perfectly, and it was a delight to enjoy. I slip down from time to time during the busy day, enjoy my rocking chair, and drink a Diet Coke. To me this rocking chair underlines the greatest joy there is in being a doctor. To be able to help someone, to be able to save a life, and to be able to be there when you are desperately needed provides one of life's greatest experiences. Oh yes, by the way, the baby is reported to be doing fine at two years of age.

Jaws!

Funeral home emergency! Can you imagine such a thing? No kidding, one of my mortuary buddies gave me a call recently. The tone of his voice indicated he really needed an emergency call at his establishment. Did the corpse show signs of life? Hardly. The problem, however, was in urgent need of a solution. The body he was preparing for showing was simply in no condition to present to the public the way it was. The mouth was wide open and the jaws were locked in the wide-open position. He did his darndest to fix the unacceptable complication but he couldn't do it. Either he missed the lecture in mortuary school in reducing a jaw dislocation or else the subject was not in the curriculum and so the frantic call from the friendly undertaker to the friendly country doctor. From his description of the problem, I pretty well figured out what the problem was. I dropped everything and drove my trusty yellow convertible Volkswagon to the funeral home. The anxious funeral director met me at the door and without further ado ushered me into the embalming room. There was my patient with his mouth wide open and his jaw dislocated and stuck. Evidently, when he suddenly experienced cardiopulmonary arrest at the hospital, the jaw was dislocated in the intubation process (inserting a breathing tube into the windpipe). For reasons unknown to me at this writing, I can't imagine this medical center hospital allowing the corpse to be removed from its premises with a dislocated jaw. But, so help me, it really happened. After death, rigor mortis sets in and muscles become very rigid and fixed.

I have reduced dislocated jaws on a few occasions in the past forty years but never on a corpse and so a new challenge. This is one of the fascinations of doctoring. One never knows what will turn up next in the run of a day. I put on my gloves and maneuvered the jaw into position. It wasn't easy, but we made it and the mouth was closed and the problem was solved. The mortician breathed a sigh of relief, a smile crossed his furrowed brow, and I knocked a home run with the bases loaded.

Had the funeral director been a Roman Catholic, I suspect he would have called the Pope on the spot and recommended that I be elevated to sainthood. How about that! St. Martin, II.

The funeral director was not sure if any kind of insurance covered the fee for a reduction of a jaw dislocation in the funeral home. I doubted if Medicare would be interested. The dead man could hardly be sent a bill. The family couldn't be told about the embarrassing incident and so, I decided that I would await my reward in the great beyond. Maybe I could use a few points on judgment day. Maybe, just maybe, the act of mercy would make up for a time or two when I had stuck my foot in my mouth. I left the funeral home a happy man. If I hadn't been able to get that wide open mouth closed, no way could the family have had a traditional open casket visitation. I had ministered to this patient many times in the previous 10 years, and on this occasion I was able to perform a service that was appreciated by the funeral director. I shall never forget that happy face as I waved goodbye.

Fox At Work

Whenever a rabid animal bites some poor soul in the county, all hell breaks loose. The patient, the family, the friends, and sometimes the community goes up in unholy smoke. The recent episode occurred one May morning when someone picked up a fox, en route to work. As the story goes, this unusually tame and pert young fox sat alongside the road. The man stopped his pickup and approached him. Mr. Fox made no attempt to vacate. Whereupon the fox was picked up and taken to work in the cab of the pickup truck. The delighted man took his prize fox into the workplace and showed him off to an admiring group of employees. Several even petted the fox. Eventually the fox was taken home and some time later it proceeded to get sick and die. Before departing, it managed to take a goodbye bite of the hand of the would-be rescuer. The bitten man thought all this a bit strange and a light flashed on in his head and he sort of got scared. He took the carcass to the local vet, who indeed advised that the head should be severed and sent to the state medical laboratory. Alas, alas, the head was positive for rabies. The victim reported to his doctor and rabies prophylactic shots were begun.

When the news reached the plant personnel, the usual hysteria erupted. Those who petted the fox insisted that saliva was all over the fox and it was reported that fox saliva dripped from the overhead of the cab of the pickup truck. The State Board of Health got tangled up in the scenario at this point and a representative appeared on the scene and proclaimed unequivocally that all those who petted the animal needed rabies shots at once. As a matter of fact they had only one day left to get them started or else. Yes, all hell broke loose, oh yes. I got calls from two men who touched the fox and wanted to start shots immediately. This all sounded a bit weird to me and I attempted to ask if the exposed had open sores or cuts. But I was given to understand that they wanted shots no matter what. I didn't think they did and when I found out that the series of shots at the county hospital would cost $1,600 per patient I was quite sure that we needed to know more before proceeding. The local doctors didn't think the men needed shots either, but the State Health Department had already pronounced judgment and so the die was cast. The hospital administrator got nervous at this point seeing perhaps $9,000 going down the financial drain without payment. I called the administrator. Then I called the local health officer. He called the State Health Department officials. I called them and it was finally settled that the shots would be paid for by the state if payment were in default at the hospital. Calm was restored on the scene. The administrator settled down. The patients were happy. The health department, I presume, was chagrined. The local health officer was mad, real mad. The workers at the factory breathed a sigh of relief. I cooled my overheated engine. The bitten man who picked up the fox was disgusted and

I suspect learned a lesson. The fox was dead. I bet no one at that factory will pick up a forlorn fox alongside the road anyway soon.

Drug Reps

I have made it a practice to see any and all drug representatives who present themselves at my office. I see them promptly as a rule. It is the way I would like to be treated were I doing their job. And, guess what, I do learn some things and occasionally a real pearl comes my way. Of course, along with that comes the expected repetition that I must listen to. But I must confess that these guys and gals who come by do a pretty good job. I am given on occasion some useful gifts along with the trivia. What's more, some real cute and pretty females come by and brighten up my visits between wheezes, coughs and snotty noses. The reps have their job cut out for them and they earn their money, in my estimation. They have much to endure and must possess patience and be able to withstand the trauma of being made to wait, or endure the indignity of rejection. Then, there are reps in the major leagues and those in the minor. I like a rep who I like! Simple as that. Some personalities you are attracted to and some you are not. Occasionally, one really turns you off. I like a rep who gets his or her point across quickly, effectively, and does not castigate his competitors too severely.

I had an experience recently that helped me to identify with reps. I walked into the gift shop of a Louisville hospital to see about marketing my new book, *Referees, Docs And God*. The gift shop manager was obviously busy and not in a good mood. Even though I introduced myself as a physician, etc. etc., she gave me no time. I was, in short, given the heave ho, a leveling influence for the high and mighty physician for sure. It was good for me, no doubt. This was not as traumatic as some indignities that I have on occasion suffered, but not real pleasant either.

The human animal is an interesting species. We love to praise and then at times we love to pound. I remember listening to a well-known surgeon, who was and is also known for his brilliance as an entertaining speaker at medical meetings. He got off the story about drug reps and it was pretty obvious that he didn't enjoy their presence at all. Said he, "The detail men who come to see me have been brain-washed. They have been lined up in the manager's office, had stomach tubes passed into their gut, and distended with lots of data. They hold it just long enough to regurgitate it in my office." Obviously, the reps who visited or attempted to visit this doctor did not in all likelihood have a happy experience. But life is like this sometimes. We all take the good with the bad and simply have to put up with a lot when we confront the public. I know; I have been there. But all in all, I would rather deal with people than I would with any other animal, especially barking dogs and rattlesnakes.

Larry

Yesterday morning the call came. Larry was going to surgery for his new heart. The long, long wait was over and the 7-hour drama was about to unfold. Larry still had many good years to give but he was running out of gas as far as his heart was concerned. He had too many heart attacks; of his six cylinders, five were shot. His previous bypass operation had bought time, but it was not enough. His waiting was done at home initially and he wore a beeper to warn him that he must stop immediately whatever he was doing and head for Indianapolis to get his transplant. He ran out of time waiting and his heart began to fail. Larry was put in the hospital at Indiana University Medical Center and could not leave until the donor heart was obtained. Strange. Praying for a heart meant someone had to die, and preferably a young person in a tragic accident.

The doctor called me today to give me the good news about my patient. The surgery was a brilliant success and all was well after the first 24 hours. The first hurdle was over and all concerned could begin to unwind just a bit. The long period of tension and uncertainty was over. The next period of waiting and uncertainty would begin soon. Would the heart function properly? Would the body reject it? Would the drugs to prevent rejection work? Would they harm? Uncertainty in every direction. During the operation the family members were gathered to comfort one another, pray and hope. The elders of the First Christian Church of Larry's home town, Salem, Indiana, quickly assembled in the chapel. Prayers and concern were the order of the day.

Sometimes at life's extremities it is companionship, love, concern that makes hell bearable. We all, if we live long enough, will have to endure pain, anxiety, frustration, and a pile of other undesirables. Most of us find the traveling easier and sometimes bearable if someone who loves us goes with us. And so Larry has been surrounded by family, friends, and those who care. It does make the difference. It does! Even at our birth we are surrounded by those who love us. During childhood, mom and dad are there for most of us. During life, in our moments of joy, we are surrounded by our companions. In sorrow likewise. Especially during illness we are comforted by those who care and at death, family, companions and friends again gather. We speculate about the great beyond. All religions have something to say about the subject. Christians look to the resurrection event and rejoice. I have a strong hunch that the God who thought all this up and planned it out is going to write our final chapter correctly. As I have submitted my body to my doctors in life, so I trust my creator to handle my affairs when I can no longer do it. It will be right. I don't have any doubt.

Say, Larry, how does it feel to have a new engine installed?

Deloris Didn't Die

She should have died, but miraculously she lived through the ordeal. "D" has been my patient for a number of years but was not seriously ill until a couple of years ago when a heart condition developed, resulting in a damaged heart valve. She was treated properly and made a good comeback. She was unable to return to her factory work but took a less stressful job in the local cap factory. Her heart condition seemed to be stabilized and life went on. One fateful day without warning she collapsed at the factory. The ambulance was summoned and the EMT's were at her side quickly. Fortunately, the factory was within sight of the hospital. The MT's found her in cardiopulmonary arrest and started CPR. She arrived at the hospital and code blue was called. CPR was still going on. No pulse, no respiration, no sign of life. In the emergency room, the team was waiting for her. The monitor revealed the fatal heart rhythm of ventricular fibrillation. The heart was shocked five times in all. On the fifth shock, the fatal rhythm was corrected to a normal sinus rhythm. There was now a faint hope. She was put on a ventilator and appropriate medications were given to resuscitate her. Her pulse gradually returned and the blood pressure began to rise. After an hour or so, she was moved to the coronary care unit at the hospital and kept there until the following day. St. Vincent's Hospital in Indianapolis was contacted and she was sent by ambulance to that facility in critical condition. Examination revealed that open heart surgery and a mitral valve replacement were necessary for her survival. The operation would be hazardous and the outcome uncertain. The family agreed and the surgery was undertaken. The valve was replaced and she made it through the risky procedure. An automatic defibrillator was put into place as well. This amazing apparatus was capable of defibrillating the heart should the fatal rhythm occur again. "D" lived through all of this and gained her strength back and is now at home, up and about, resuming her life.

This is a beautiful example of team work. The MT's are to be given much credit for saving her life. The marvels of medical advancement is evident here. The brilliance of our surgical expertise is demonstrated. "D" is alive. Thank God.

Pop-Tarts And Pap Tests

Pop-Tarts are good. The kids love them and so do moms and dads. Those good, cripsy, fruity flavored, wafers of joy that we toast at breakfast are delicious. But pap tests are for the birds. I mean women hate them. Why? Lots of reasons. First of all, you might find out that you have something wrong with you and that is pretty upsetting. But if you want your birth control pill prescription renewed, you have to get your pap test. You have to make an appointment with the doctor, wait in the office too long, then get on that wretched exam table, expose yourself in a most embarrassing position and endure some possible discomfort during the procedure. Cold instruments to boot. You have to pay for all this trouble and then sometimes you get a report that there are some bad cells and a biopsy is necessary. This is more time, more trouble, more exposure, and more money, and maybe more bad news. Pap tests are indeed for the birds. If a man had to have one, there wouldn't be any done, more than likely.

Now I have heard some very interesting comments as women speak their mind (about the time the sheet is draped and the speculum inserted.) Mostly it's mutterings to the effect that, "I'd rather take a beating than get this done." One woman went so far as to say that she'd rather have a baby than go through this. Now that comment was about the ultimate. "Doc, you don't know how I hate this," is a favorite remark. Well, that's true. I don't know. I guess I wouldn't be real thrilled to have a female doctor perform a vasectomy on me, come to think about it.

Which brings up another interesting matter. Docs rarely go to a doctor unless it is life or death. We typically treat ourselves. We don't have time, the desire, or the courage to go to a doctor. We get sick in one way or another, grab some pills and hope for the best. There is the old saying and maybe it is true. The doctor who doctors himself has a damn fool for a doctor. Nevertheless, the majority of doctors don't have a family doctor, a favorite psychiatrist, or whatever. We get sick and finally decide we have to get some advice. We make rounds at the hospital. We spy our favorite urologist in the hallway and ask him to step into the bathroom and check us. The prostate is bad, real bad. He comes in and you thrust a glove and some lubricating jelly into his hand and he checks your prostate gland, gives you some advice, and you try to carry it out. No notes, no nothing. A lousy way to practice medicine but that is the way it is done. Doctors still are taken to surgery to have their appendix taken out, but they may well have delayed the examination until the abscess or rupture has occurred.

The Great Dane at our house one day stretched himself out on our couch and occupied the entire space. I repeatedly requested politely that he remove himself. When he saw fit not to do that, I hit him over his back side with my fist and fractured my fifth metacarpal over his lumbar spinous process. Did I see a doc? No! I got the x-ray all right but I didn't have the time or the inclination to have a cast put on so I wrapped it up and went about my work as best I could. Did it hurt? You bet it did! Good treatment. Real good.

Doctors, when they are patients in hospitals, can be a disaster to all in attendance. They obviously know too much, question too much, talk too much and generally are not favorite people to care for, but many do get sick, and by the grace of God, a few get well despite it all.

Doctor Bills

The current doctor-patient relationship deterioration is evident about everywhere and I don't think anyone likes it (except for some lawyers.) I am certain that the lawyers who specialize in malpractice cases are thrilled. It is like finding a new fishing hole where the big fish are. Certainly I don't like the position of failing rapport between doctors and patients, and I am sure the patients don't like it either. You and your doctor may be getting along very well indeed and there is no problem. I hope that is the case. But on the whole, it is generally agreed that doctor-patient relationships are not as good as they were 50 or even 25 years ago. Why? The reasons are multiple but one of them is due to the high cost of medical care. People just hate to pay medical bills. No bills are popular come to think about it. I am not actually thrilled to pay $10,000 to Washington County for real estate taxes this year either and I have never been thrilled to give a large chunk of my income to the IRS. Nor have I always enjoyed paying my malpractice insurance premiums.

But medical bills are especially onerous to pay. We don't want to be sick in the first place and then to have to pay to get well is plain terrible. We buy a new car and don't seem to mind that bill much or a new house or whatever, but to pay because you get sick is just for the birds. I can relate to that. Paying a few thousand dollars over and above my insurance to doctors and hospitals a few years ago when I had my last hospitalization was not a joyful experience I can assure you. But I am glad I did it and I am grateful to be well.

Here is how I view the situation of run away health care expense:

1. The general public believes that doctors charge entirely too much and therefore overcharging is the cause of the problem. I must regretfully confess that I believe this to be true often. However, I believe overcharging to be only the tip of the iceberg.

2. America can and does provide the best health care in the world but the expense has become prohibitive for many. We have highly trained doctors who usually are well qualified and often are highly intelligent, dedicated, and skilled at what they do. We have the best hospitals in the world. Most of us have ready access to hospital care and procedures. We are utilizing high technology as never before. Cosmetic surgery, transplants and bypasses, pacemakers, are routine. But all of this is very very expensive. People live longer and longer resulting in more and more expense as people require more and more care. It is a vicious cycle. Keeping *dead* people alive creates an expense of alarming proportions.

3. If we are successful in our efforts to control the cost of health care and provide universal health care to our people, then we Americans will have to accept the situation quite different from what it is today. Some Americans are proposing a tax-supported universal government-controlled health care system. We will not like, however, the inevitable rationing of care, the de-personalization in the system, the waiting that will have to be a part of the system and endure many of the other economy measures that we are not presently used to. Finally, if the practice of medicine of tomorrow is such that doctors and other health care people do not consider the rewards commensurate with their investment, then we will not get quality people to work in the health care field. That inevitably brings about a reduction in the standard of health care.

Tidbits For Young Doctors

1. Don't make your doctor angry. I want a happy doctor working on me.

2. Be careful in choosing your words, the patient did not go to medical school.

3. Be careful about the words you use. You may unnecessarily scare someone.

4. If you can't help the patient, don't hurt him.

5. It takes a special breed of woman to live with a doctor; may God help her. And it takes a special breed of man to live with a high-powered, professional female.

6. Two hundred years ago on the American frontier, the pioneer feared the Indian, disease and the elements. Now we fear mugging, the court room and AIDS.

7. "I know I shouldn't be calling at 2 in the morning, Doc, but it's me."

8. At the University Hospital the LMD (local medical doctor) is often regarded as a second-class citizen. The big shots are vital in the war against disease and injury, but so are the little shots out there where the bullets fly and the blood flows.

9. Death and taxes are inevitable and there are certain things a doctor simply has to accept and put up with, such as failures and frustrations. He must recognize that some things and some people can't be fixed.

10. The media with a little knowledge and an ax to grind can be a monster to the doctor. I have to spend lots of time untying the knots that the media ties around the doctor's leg. Happily, sometimes the media is very helpful.

11. We appreciate our ears when we are going deaf and we value our eyes when we are going blind.

12. When a surgeon does his first operation, I am not sure who is the most nervous, the doc or the patient.

13. Doctor, if you score a medical hole in one, you just might be praised, but if you cut off the wrong leg, you are sure to be sued.

14. You can be dreadfully sick if you think you are. Likewise, sometimes you can recover from an illness by believing you are well.

15. We admire the person who has the potential to make a million dollars, but decides rather to give his energy for a great cause and live frugally.

16. When it is mandatory to face a life or death decision, it is a comforting experience to place your life into the care of a doctor you trust completely.

17. The roots and herbs in the doctor's office one hundred years ago didn't accomplish much. They didn't hurt either, and the placebo effect was often helpful. Modern drugs can work miracles; they also can kill. Use them with caution.

18. When a mistake is made, it is easy to put someone down. It is more difficult and challenging to suggest that there might be a better way.

19. No man prefers to have his prostate checked because it involves a rectal exam. The doctor doesn't especially enjoy it either, but I would rather be the doctor than the patient.

20. We may argue all day and night about a supernatural devil. There is no argument, however, that plenty of natural devils are alive and well.

21. Most of us hate to be sick, but a few souls apparently refuse to be well.

22. Why is it that the fat can't get skinny, and the skinny can't get fat? I guess it was meant to be that way?

23. Tough decision: When to insist on your own way and when to yield to the other guy.

24. Tough decision: When to treat the case medically or surgically.

25. Tough decision: Whether to allow death with dignity or to continue life at any cost.

26. Tough decision: Tell the truth and nothing but the truth or hedge just a little.

27. Tough decision: To marry or not to marry.

28. Very tough decision: Yes or no.

29. If you like your job, it's a blessing many don't have. As a matter of fact, if you have any job, you are blessed.

30. The primary doctor is doing few procedures, making fewer decisions, being assisted by every Tom, Dick and Harry, and told what to do and what not to do, and generally is relegated to a lower rung on the ladder. Nevertheless, he is asked to sign the bottom line, taking full responsibility for the entire ballgame.

31. When the critics of the medical establishment get real sick, they generally go to the nearest emergency room for help.

32. Psychiatry is often regarded as a second rate stepchild of medicine until the patient bites the nurse, sits on the aid, kicks the doctors and throws the bedpan against the wall. For the moment the stepchild is respected.

33. Hospital personnel generally don't like the Behavioral Medicine Unit but tolerate it because it may keep the hospital from bankruptcy. When a patient is on Med-Surg and goes berserk, BMU is suddenly appreciated.

34. Don't condemn your colleague in front of the patient: you wouldn't enjoy that either.

35. Listen carefully and attentively to your patients. You'll learn things and you'll be a good doctor.

36. Don't have unrealistic expectations from your patients. Most are unwilling to change their lifestyle in order to assist in their recovery.

37. A few will stop drinking to excess.

38. A few will stop smoking.

39. Slow down. Tomorrow is another day. This too will pass. You may be tired, but remember, the patient is likely scared.

40. Beware of the patient who overdoes it with compliments. He may ask for the moon before he leaves.

41. Remember, the patient may not have read the medical book before he got sick.

42. Treat the patient, not the x-ray or the lab report.

43. Don't forget the bowels as you study the monitor.

44. There are times when life is worse than death.

45. It is a dreadful thing to have to perform an abortion. But it is likewise a dreadful thing to grow up unloved and unwanted.

46. Treatment for vomiting: a quick emesis basin.

47. Nursing home existence is just that, but it beats the street.

48. Keep a closed mind; otherwise, you might have to change it.

49. Resist the temptation to preach; it is a waste of time.

50. Some people want to be sick. The sooner you discover that the better.

51. The candidate for an insurance policy looks great, acts great and is great. The candidate for a disability exam may look bad, act bad and be bad.

52. Some people want to be hugged — go ahead, and give them a break.

53. Until a lawsuit is settled, the patient will continue to complain.

54. Doctoring is stressful, but being the patient is worse.

55. We have instant food but not instant health.

56. Some insist on shots while others refuse them.

57. When the patient is ill or injured on his own time, he runs back to work. When on company time, he crawls back to work.

58. The doctor who doctors himself has a damn fool for a doctor. This includes about all of us.

Medical Problems That Doctor's Don't Like

There are two problems that are prevalent in every primary doctor's practice that are really difficult for all concerned. If you are afflicted with chronic headache or chronic backache, may the Lord above pity you. No one else does. The doctor is frustrated because he simply doesn't have the tools to handle chronic headache and backache very well. The patient is frustrated because he can't get sympathy or relief. Of course, there are exceptions to the rule and at times we docs zero in on the cause of headache or backache and bring about relief.

The patient with chronic emotional problems and or chronic pain problems presents a burden to all concerned. The patient suffers and so do those around the patient. The spouse and significant others in the patient's life pay a price to continue the relationship. The doctor, who really tries to help, takes on a great big burden. Sometimes it is really hard to know what is in the best interest of all concerned. The struggle that erupts once habituating drugs and narcotics are utilized is often a heavy burden for all concerned.

A patient with multiple complaints that have an emotional origin is especially difficult. So often the patient refuses to accept the diagnosis and wanders from doctor to doctor in search of relief. That often does not easily come. Often the patient becomes the victim of multiple drug dependence which is obviously not in anyone's best interest.

Then there is the drug seeker who makes the rounds in search of habituating medications and often tells a convincing story in an attempt to justify his request. These people have serious problems and need attention, but usually are not aware of their problems. If they are, they are usually unwilling to come to grips with the situation.

Doctor's Hit Parade

1. Peer Review.
2. Medicare.
3. Medicaid.
4. Second opinion.
5. Mandated by the government.
6. Do it or suffer the consequences.
7. "Have your doctor fill out this form for you (four pages)."
8. We want your total health history.
9. "Have your doctor send this form to us at no expense to us."
10. "I don't want to cause trouble, but because I have suffered so much from an unnecessary operation, I feel compelled to seek compensation for the doctor's negligence." In other words, a greenback poultice is demanded.

Medical Doctors The Patient's Don't Like

A good doctor-patient relationship is a grand thing. A bad one is bad. Just like a marriage in a way. Some patients want a doctor who is laid back, relaxed, takes his time, visits with his patient, and generally is not in a hurry. If this patient ends up with a doctor who is always in a hurry, zips in and out of the room before you see the color of his shirt, then a problem arises.

There are authoritative doctors who give out orders without explanation. This just doesn't go over very well with the inquisitive patient who wants answers. There are physicians whose fees are outrageously high and this is reflected in a lifestyle that is likewise a bit outrageous. This sort of situation gives medicine a black eye in my opinion and is hastening the day when third parties and government take full control of medical practice. And then, of course, there is the doctor who is cold and detached which often creates a problem. The patient may get the message that the doctor is unconcerned when actually he is. It's simply a matter of personality and should not be taken personally. Some patients want doctors whose style permits the patient to participate in the medical scene. Others want a doctor who does all the leading and commanding and leaves no decision with the patient. Problems arise consequently when a round hole is approached by a square plug.

Of course it would be nice if all doctors could be brilliant, dedicated, have a warm and pleasant personality, charge reasonable fees, and adopt a decent lifestyle. Seldom do we find all these qualities resident in any one doctor. The same can be said of patients. Seldom do we find the perfect patient, that is, one who follows instructions, keeps appointments, does his part in bringing about the healing process, is appreciative, pays his bills, and tells the world that he has a great doctor. Life just isn't that way. We do the best, or try to, with what we have and let the chips fall.

The Patient's Hit Parade

1. Payment is expected at the receipt of service unless prior arrangements have been made.

2. Your appointment is at 2 o'clock, actually you are seen at 3:30.

3. "Take two aspirin and call me in the morning."

4. "Doctor, explain to me what you plan to do." "Trust me, that is all you need to do."

5. "Doctor, do you think a chiropractor could help?" Blank stare of hurtful disbelief from the doctor.

6. "There is nothing the matter with you." This is said with the patient holding his chest with trembling hands.

7. "It only took 45 minutes and he charged me $1,000."

8. "I have spent $5,000 and they still don't know what my trouble is."

9. "The baby was born in bed ten minutes after they told me to calm down because I was not ready for delivery."

10. "The doctor said it is all in my head and I know damn good and well that it isn't."

11. "They say it used to be quiet in the hospital but now it is the noisiest place in town."

12. "He said it would only hurt a little."

13. "I'll be there in just a minute."

14. "I think you need to see a psychiatrist."

15. "Stop smoking and your cold will improve."

16. "You need to lose 50 pounds of weight."

17. "Just relax and you can sleep. You don't need a pill."

18. "Stop your drinking or your liver will get you."

19. "Your weight gain, my dear, is not due to fluid."

20. "You say you can't fasten your pants anymore. No, it is not due to gas."

Three Cheers For The Media

I didn't think I would ever live to see the day when TV did it right from the viewpoint of the doctor. But last night on the MacNeil Lehrer Report, they did it right and I hasten to congratulate them. It is obvious that when someone takes our side of an argument we think they are great. It is just human nature. So often I have felt the media has done the doctor and the health care delivery system a disservice by the reporting of everything imaginable wrong with the way medical care is dispensed. So often it seems we are clobbered by what is perceived as our deficiencies and failures and little is said about all the great things that are accomplished. Be that as it may, last night the media did it right. I want to stand up and cheer.

Health care costs are out of control. Upon this premise there is no debate. The question is, "Why is this true and what can be done about it?" There were two important points brought out by the media and I can't agree more with the emphasis. This is crucial. Americans demand the best when it comes to health care and generally get it. We have high tech in about every field and the best that medical care can deliver. We can do a great deal for sick people that was unheard of 50 years ago. But all this comes at a very high price. And to make matters worse, we want someone else to pay for our medical care.

We simply can't have our cake and eat it too. Either we will have to reduce our expectations or we will have to continue to pay more and more as advances are made in the medical field. One is tempted to say "Let the government take over the system and cost containment will come." I will agree that there is presently a lot of waste in the system and there are many ways that we could save money by restructuring the medical care delivery system. Nevertheless, if we cost-contain, then we will get what we pay for and no more. There are no bargain basement prices in the business of life or death.

And so, is there an answer? There are some things that can be better. Here are a few suggestions from a doctor who has been out there where the action is for about 50 years.

1. If your doctor says that MRI is really not necessary, please don't insist on it. It costs somebody $1,000 or more.

2. Use emergency services only in case of true emergencies.

3. Don't sue your doctor for every mistake. He is not perfect. Only God is.

4. Be willing to accept rationing of medical services when it becomes necessary.

5. Be willing to let loved ones die with dignity and do not insist on continuing life at whatever the cost if there is no quality of life left.

6. American's can prevent illness and injury if they will do the following. Don't drink and drive, quit smoking, drive safely, don't eat so much.

7. Remember, if you don't take care of your body, your repair bill will be astronomical, just like your automobile if you treat it with disrespect.

Free At Last

This statement we all recognize as the one made by the immortal Martin Luther King, Jr. Today I feel that I can make this statement without reservation. Yes, Yes, Yes! Free at last I am. On Thursday, the 12th of July, the hangman's noose was removed from my neck and I walked down from the gallows. It is a wonderful feeling I can tell you that. For three years I have lived with a malpractice lawsuit at my doorstep. I was accused of negligence in failing to diagnose soon enough to save a life. Finally, the day for the panel to meet was scheduled. The panel consisted of three doctors and one lawyer. They were given copies of the medical records and the copies of the allegations brought against me along with my defense. The panel convened and discussed the case. I was given the opportunity to attend the meeting and listen only. The attorneys and I went into the conference room at the appropriate time. The plaintiff attorney asked several questions, each one designed to show some form of negligence on my part. On each occasion the doctors took my side and defended my actions as appropriate. They indicated that I had done a pretty good job considering the fact that I was seeing a vast number of patients and bearing an exceedingly heavy load in my practice. Clearly, I was exonerated. The plaintiff attorney said to my attorney in my presence afterwards that he had no case and would recommend that the case be dropped. The marvelous relief that this brought is known only to those who have walked the path. It is a tremendous burden removed, the feeling of which is indescribably sweet. Free at last, yes, free at last!

Night

Problems always seem to be worse at night. No question. A critical patient in the coronary care unit and I have to make an important decision. It is tough at night. Obstructed labor and the baby in difficulty. It's 2 o'clock in the morning and it is a lot tougher than at 2 o'clock in the afternoon. At least that is the way it is with me. It seems at night that you are alone with your stress and decision-making. When the sun is up you have companionship. It is easier to face the enemy when you have company. But nights have to follow day and we have to do what we have to do. Nights can be great when we can sleep undisturbed and get up refreshed and rearing to go. But in the 40 years of hospital and office practice, I, like all doctors, have spent many a night working instead of sleeping.

Night has come to my life on an extended basis several times and it has to all of us of course. Three trips to a psychiatric facility struggling with depression has meant the blackest of night for weeks at a time. Night has come to our lives over and over as we have given up loved ones. Night comes when a child is in surgery and the outcome is uncertain. Night has come to my friend, Dave, when he gave up his wife recently with cancer.

But, thank God, morning does follow night and we gain our equilibrium and our motivation. Sunsets are gorgeous but I somehow like sunrise the best.

Media Monster

I have just turned off the television. They have launched another attack on a good drug and no doubt others will pick up the war cry and try to ruin its reputation. Oh yes, I am for freedom of the media all right, but this liberty can and does do untold damage to the innocent sometimes, be it drugs, merchandise, insecticides, or people. Tonight, the commentator chose to clobber an excellent drug called Xanax. Just like the press killed Valium, an excellent drug, when properly used. But it was hounded to death and as a result, if a doctor elects to use it he has to slip it across and use a generic equivalent name on the prescription. Why? If the patient saw the name Valium written on the prescription, he might think the doctor was incompetent because of the bad press that Valium has been given. The press knows better than all the doctors, of course they do. And so tonight I had to listen to the case against Xanax. Sure, some people become addicted. But think of the blessings it has brought to suffering patients. No mention of that whatsoever. Fifty-thousand people will be killed by automobiles this year and millions injured. Why not get rid of automobiles and go to horses! About the same logic as this Xanax attack! It's not the cars' fault that 50,000 people are killed and millions injured. It's the drivers' fault, for goodness sakes! Xanax is not at fault, it's the patient who is addiction-prone. Xanax may have withdrawal problems but they can be dealt with. But tell me, is there a perfect drug anywhere? Oh yes, some psychiatrists get in the act and claim that Xanax is a curse of Satan. The trouble is the psychiatrist mainly sees the addicted people and not the thousands who are helped by Xanax. Yes, Xanax has been dealt a severe blow by the most powerful persuader the earth has ever been blessed with, namely television. I will have to spend hours defending my use of Xanax because of television's delightful presentation showing only one side of a situation. A verdict will be made after the prosecutor sits down and the defense has not had even a chance to open its mouth. That is not fair. That is not right. That is for the birds. Why not attack penicillin? A hundred people will die this year from allergic reactions from penicillin and many may suffer non-fatal reactions. Why not attack aspirin? Many will develop ulcers, a few will bleed and some will perhaps have a near death, if not a death experience because of aspirin. The media does not seem to get too upset about cigarettes and whiskey and we know the death and destruction brought about by these products.

If I were an executive of the Upjohn Pharmaceutical Firm, I would be extremely upset tonight and with good reason. They had no chance to defend their product, but the media and their personnel have chosen to play doctor and inform all of us how we should practice and what we should do. They obviously know more than all doctors and all pharmaceutical people know about Xanax and most certainly they know more than the lowly country doctor who is out in the trenches trying to relieve suffering humanity.

It's Not Fun To Be Sick

I have had two pretty good days in my current struggle with a disgusting malady. Chronic recurrent bacterial prostatitus it is called. Yes, I said disgusting. In the first place, once you get it, you can never really get rid of the darn stuff. It keeps coming back, like trying to get rid of the flies in the kitchen. The prostate gland is such a lowly organ, seemingly not all that important, and sort of a private part of your body that you don't go around talking about. Not like the glorious heart, which when it is subjected to a quadruple bypass, causes us to rip open our shirts and show our scar and tell the world about our new-found life and resurrection from the grave. Just the old beat up prostate, almost ignominious, and unworthy of discussion in public. To tell you the truth, the prostate is pretty important to the average male at all ages beyond puberty.

For the sexually active male, it is vital. It produces a secretion which is an important component of the seminal fluid. Now I can tell you for sure that most males tend to regard that as a vitally important function but not the subject of public discussion. The prostate is mighty important to the older men too. Often it continues to grow when every other part of the body is shrinking. And what happens? Some morning, the victim of this condition gets up and goes to the bathroom for his morning initial activity, and low and behold he can't pee a drop. Absolutely, positively, he is in terrible shape and to the emergency room at the local hospital he goes in a hurry. He feels like he is in the last stages of labor and he is begging for mercy. At the emergency room the young doc on duty slips in the catheter to relieve him and let me tell you, this procedure is not a piece of cake. Quite frankly, it can hurt real bad, and usually does. But it brings wonderful, oh so glorious, relief. I guess like having a baby.

But back to my favorite malady, recurrent bacterial prostatitis. I have wrestled with this disgusting disease for 15 years and I am flat out sick and tired of it. You simply can't get over it and know you are over it, never to return, like good old chicken pox. This present attack has been on me for six weeks. Initially, one has chills and fever and feels like he has a coal of fire in his rectum. You have an urgency to go to the bathroom every few minutes and when you get the signal to go, you better not delay or you will be sorry. I usually at this point reach on my medicine shelf and select an antibiotic and after a week of taking it I feel good. But not this last time. By grabs, I have used six antibiotics in all and maybe, just maybe, this last one is going to put out the fire. Every day I am dragging, my energy is gone, and I have aches and pains all over. I don't want to do much more than I have to. My body yearns to lie down and let the world go by. I hate that. I am a man of action and I hate to wait for healing to occur, like so many of my patients. At one stretch I took an antibiotic by injection, 10 in the right butt and 10 in the left one and as a result I am black and blue and sore and prefer to stand up.

Yes, I hate to be sick. I would so much rather be a doctor than a patient. It is a dangerous job to be a doctor anymore, with a lawyer circling overhead awaiting a kill, but it is worse to be a patient with the undertaker circling around waiting for a call.

Heparin And Hope

On this first day of spring, I am lying propped up in bed in the hospital impatiently awaiting the clot in my left leg vein to stabilize and the inflammation to subside. We Americans are an impatient lot, and I suspect doctors are some of the worst. As a matter of fact, I know so. My sentence is for a week's stay in the hospital receiving heparin in my vein. Heparin is an anti-coagulant that is frequently used to prevent clot formation under a number of circumstances. A clot in the leg vein causes pain, tenderness and swelling, and creates the potential for complications. If a person has a clot break loose from the vein, it will go to the heart and on to the lung and cause immediate chest pain and possibly death. Therefore, it is no joking matter but must be regarded as a real threat.

All this developed three days before I consulted the doctor. I knew what the trouble was and started my own treatment. I tried to avoid the hospital for obvious reasons, but to no avail. I was forced by my constituency to do what I didn't want to do. And so, with reluctance, I saw my doctor, had testing done to check me for clots by a high tech machine, and received the verdict. A clot was in the leg and a week in the hospital would be required to deal with it.

At this writing, I have endured four days of my seven-day sentence. I have to confess, it could be a lot worse. No pain pills, no sleeping pills, only a continuous drip of that magic clot inhibiting juice known as heparin going into my vein 24-hours a day.

As memory serves me, the idea of anti-coagulant drugs was learned from the secrets of the leech. That little animal heparinizes his victim in order to suck out the blood and keep it in a liquid state.

I feel like a race horse locked up in a barn. I think most busy people feel that way when subjected to a hospital stay. But I realize perhaps better than most people that things could be far worse. I don't have the sentence of death upon me. I have hope of recovery. No cancer. No stroke. Not even major surgery.

Forty-six years ago I was a medical student across the street from Norton Hospital where I now am. The Louisville General Hospital, where all medical students cut their eye teeth, was a big, big place. The buildings were spread out and not so high as they now are. The changes on the inside of the hospital were even more dramatic. Here we have private rooms, nicely furnished, with bath and TV for all. In 1946, at Louisville General Hospital, big open wards for 30 patients were utilized instead of private rooms and there was no TV and no private anything. Lives were saved then but not to compare with the salvage today.

I select my menu and usually get what I ask for. The service is good and my stay is made as painless as possible.

Doctors are not usually the most popular patients on the nurse's list. They know too much, question too much and generally can and often do act like jerks. I really try to behave. I try to take orders, say thanks, don't moan and groan and complain unless compelled to do so. I don't ask for the moon and try to fit in with the landscape. I try to smile and be pleasant. Service is apt to be correspondingly given with a smile. If I had cancer, leukemia or was totally paralyzed, I suspect I would be struggling with depression and anger. We can't always avoid disaster, tragedy or intense suffering, but we do have some control about a reaction to misfortune. We don't have to be miserable and make everyone who comes in to see us miserable, or do we?

From Stab Wound To Transplant

In 1946 open heart surgery was unheard of. It was impossible to bypass the heart using the heart-lung machine. Such technology was not even on the drawing board. The nearest thing to open heart surgery was carried out one night when a man was stabbed in the heart but was still alive although in deep shock. When he arrived at the Louisville General Hospital Emergency Room, it was evident after X-rays that he had a cardiac tamponade (blood surrounding the heart within the pericardial sac). The pressure of the blood was restricting the pump action critically and death was imminent. He was then taken to surgery, put to sleep, and the chest cavity opened. The heart was exposed and the bulging sac (pericardium) was exposed. It was opened, blood sucked out, and the hole in the heart identified by the geyser of blood that squirted each time the heart beat. The surgeon's finger was placed over the hole and three sutures were taken in the incision, closing the defect, and all was well.

Within a short time a technique was worked out to relieve mitral stenosis. This is a situation in which a heart valve is narrowed critically from disease resulting in a failing heart and eventual death of the patient. It was discovered that a surgeon could expose the heart, open one of the heart chambers, and insert his index finger and open up the defect allowing the damned up blood in the lungs to flow freely. It was known as the *finger fracture procedure* for relieving mitral stenosis. This too could be done with the heart beating and without bypassing the heart and lungs.

In the early 1960's I attended a medical meeting at the Lexington Clinic, Lexington, Kentucky. I have attended many but this one stands out above all the rest. A doctor by the name of Soones from Cleveland Clinic gave a lecture about a revolutionary idea to attack the problem of coronary stenosis (blockage of the heart arteries). This condition was the leading cause of death in the United States and still is. He developed a technique for visualizing the blood flow through the coronary arteries and then identifying the areas of obstruction. It was called cardiac catheterization. We sat on the edge of our seats in silence and looked and listened to the presenter knowing that we were witnessing a new era in surgery. A patient had to go to Cleveland then for his open heart surgery. A pump and an oxygenator were devised for a mechanical substitute for the heart and lungs. This made it possible to bypass the heart and lungs, stop the heart, and suture in place veins taken from the leg of the patient. The vein would then act as a detour for the blood to flow around the obstruction in the coronary artery. This procedure, done only at first in Cleveland, is now done in every city of any size in the United States. Thousands are improving their quality of life as well as extending their life span because of this procedure. Now finally it is possible to transplant another human heart into a patient when the heart is worn out completely. Unbelievable but true. Fifty years ago the chest was rarely opened for any operation.

Where do we go from here? As people grow older, debilitating problems of arthritis, dementia, and strokes make for a very poor quality of life despite its increased length. If as much progress could be made in enabling mankind to live together in peace as we are in extending the life spans, we would really ring the bell for mankind.

Dementia

Dementia simply means a condition of failing intellect. It is especially to be feared by aging people. Many nursing home residents are demented. Dementia is often the reason for their admission. It is a malady to be feared for a number of reasons. There is no treatment, no reversal of the process, and usually it only gets worse with time. The aged population is increasing rapidly as medical and surgical therapy is improved. The problem intensifies accordingly.

The form of dementia known as Alzheimer's Disease is accompanied by death of brain cells for reasons unknown. It can be seen in various degrees and in various stages. There are demented people who can live a fairly decent lifestyle with minimal if any supervision. Others are so far advanced that they descend into an infantile state. My own father lay in bed in the nursing home three years. He was mute and incontinent. He was fed until death mercifully took him away.

As in all medical conditions for which there is no cure, there are many remedies that are offered for sale by the honest and by the dishonest. There is no effective and legitimate treatment for dementia except in only a select few. The usual cases of dementia are due to Alzheimer's Disease, or to strokes. The dementia caused by B12 deficiency or folic acid deficiency is treatable. Dementia from alcoholism is treatable if a person can and will stop drinking.

In all ages of life there are stresses that are peculiar to that age. Children and youth have stresses that the elderly don't have and vice versa. The elderly worry about aches and pains, failing health, dependency, and the prospect of a nursing home existence. Young people worry about their future, success or failure, finding their niche in life, peer pressure, and leaving the nest.

I have seen a few examples in which dementia has actually benefited the patient. A few patients at the nursing home find their initial adjustment impossible and they become bitter, angry, complaining, and make themselves and all around them miserable. When dementia creeps over them, they slowly mellow out and become a kitty cat instead of a tiger.

United States Of America Health Care Dilemma 1993

From a country doctor's point of view and after 45 years of practice, I'll toss in the ring some thoughts about health care in the USA. Of all the problems that we face in America, and there are many, this one rates high on our priority list. The economy, drug dependence, AIDS, crime, national debt, the homeless, and the search for peace of mind despite our abundance indicates that health care is not our only problem by any means. And then too, we are disturbed about our legal climate in which we are battling each other in the courtroom at an unprecedented rate. It is to the lawyers' delight but to the disadvantage of the rest of us.

It is interesting to note that despite our dilemmas about health care, patients and doctors from all over the world continue to come to America to be a part of the medical scene. We have the best of all things in health care if we can afford it, and that is the heart of the problem. Can we afford to have services that we demand, and how can we make the services available to all who want and deserve them? Is health care a right or a privilege? No ready answers here.

Is it best to have fee-for-service health care or salaried health care? Human nature being what it is, the salaried physician is tempted not to work so hard and the fee-for-service physician may work to an excess. That usually means some procedures are done that are not absolutely necessary. The salaried physician on the other hand may not do some procedures that are indicated. So what is best?

If we are to control costs then we will have to accept the economy package. If you want a less expensive automobile, you can't have deluxe features and likewise with health care. To make health care available to all and to give basic health care needs to all will mean the following:

1. There inevitably must be some sort of rationing of health care. Everyone cannot have everything. Basic health care should be available to all and in order to do this, high cost cannot be avoided. Deluxe health care cannot be given to all. If you can afford the deluxe then okay but, if not, you cannot have it.

2. Dying with dignity must be accepted by Americans if we are to control the cost. Millions of health care dollars are

spent in keeping *dead people* alive in our nursing homes. To die with dignity is not yet allowed. But it must be. Someday we will look back on this day where we see death with indignity as a sad day and ask ourselves "How could we have done it?"

3. The responsibility for shaping the future of the medical delivery system should rest with government and other third parties, the public and the medical establishment. All of these must have input into the process. This balance of power will be difficult to achieve but represents the ideal approach. If there is great unhappiness in any of these three power bases over the evolved system, then we'll have lots of trouble.

4. When in due time we shall have arrived at a more acceptable method of health care delivery in the United States we likely will have to accept the following developments.

Doctors will continue to endure bureaucracy and third party power, rules and regulations that will sometimes be unnecessary and destructive to morale. Medical care will be rationed. Not everyone can receive the best and the most ideal treatment. Patients will wait for procedures and for surgical intervention and there will be inconvenience not to mention the occasional disaster that will occur because of delay. Beautiful, modern hospitals and doctor's offices will gradually pass from the scene as we have to accept the old and out-of-date along with the new. Doctor-patient relationships will change. The patient will be attached to a clinic, or HMO instead of the family doctor. The personal touch will give way to the institutionalized attachment. Malpractice chaos will likely improve. Patients will direct their anger and frustration at the government and third parties rather than at the doctor who currently is taking the beating. As tax dollars pay more for medical care and doctors make less money, the public will not be as angry as they are now toward the medical profession. Multiple schemes to pattern our health care delivery system have been proposed. I am not smart enough or knowledgeable enough to propose a program that will be ideal. I don't think there is any. Whatever comes out in the wash will be a compromise, the three constituents, government, other third parties, the public and the doctors, will have to abide by a less-than-ideal situation. Hopefully, it will be better than we now know. If the practice of medicine becomes difficult and unrewarding in the new scheme of things, then the quality of medical care will deteriorate as fewer qualified men and women select a health care career. Conversely, if we want top flight people to select a medical career, then the rewards will have to be commensurate.

Aunt Mary

Recently I attended the funeral service for this dear lady. She was the wife of my Uncle Wallace Cauble. I had the responsibility and the privilege of seeing that her last days on earth were made as comfortable as possible and to guide and help the family cope with her care. She died at home tenderly and expertly cared for by her caregivers. She died with dignity and we did not have to prolong the dying process. This was made possible because we elected to keep her at home where we were able to make comfort our goal and not simply the prolongation of life at any cost. Aunt Mary enjoyed good health until a few years before death when she became a victim of Alzheimer's Disease. She advanced from the early manifestations of mild memory loss to the full blown picture of confusion and disorientation. Later she developed congestive heart failure and this was successfully treated. Sometimes she was confused, combative and her behavior was controlled with medication. She lost her appetite and failed rapidly. Soon, mercifully, she left us and went to her reward peacefully. To me, this represents a scenario in which I rejoice and wish more could exit this world in this fashion. Her suffering was not prolonged, the family was not depleted of strength and morale, and her delivery to a better world was allowed to proceed without our artificial intervention. To me this is the way it should be, could be and hopefully will be for all people someday.

Unfortunately, so many of our sick and dying are subjected to the indignities of prolonging the dying process. Most die in an institution. Because of current rules, regulations, laws, codes of ethic, family wishes, we do not allow people to die naturally. To the contrary, in our nursing homes, many people without any quality of life whatsoever, are kept alive in all sorts of life-prolonging efforts. People who are in a vegetative state are fed artificially by stomach tube and cared for like a baby. When an acute medical complication arises, often the patient goes to a hospital, and more effort is spent prolonging an existence but not a life. Medical efforts spent in this fashion could and should be spent where it could help the most. I refer to those who have no medical insurance, and to children who are medically neglected for economic reasons. I long for, pray for, hope for, the day when sanity can rule our decision process and humaneness be our watchword as we minister to those who are helpless. We take great pride in our medical accomplishments to make birth safe and secure. Let us remember that we also have a responsibility to allow the terminally ill and those without any quality of life to die with dignity.

Tidbits For Young Doctors

1. I borrowed $40,000 to get started in my practice. Now doctors are wooed into the community and the road is paved with gold, so to speak. This seems sweet, but doctor, you must not expect all your roads to be likewise paved.

2. Surgeons earn more than medical doctors. Having done surgery myself, I would agree that a surgeon's life is perhaps more stressful than others. Nevertheless, unless the pay gap is narrowed sufficiently, we will not get primary doctors out on the front lines.

3. Sunrise and sunsets are similar and so is infancy and senility.

4. Doctor Bodine Stalker of Borden, Indiana, is said to have been one of the first in the long ago to get a Model T car. He made lots of house calls and, despite the muddy roads, thought this would make life easier for him. He returned one morning to town and stopped by the train depot where a couple of citizens were gathered. He had delivered a poor woman of her baby and he had been up all night and was paid nothing. Returning to town he got stuck in the mud and he had to be unceremoniously pulled out by a team of horses. When he arrived in town he was tired and muddy and disgusted. Said he, "There are only two kinds of people that drive a Model T car in Borden. One of them is a rich man and the other is a fool, and I am sure not the rich man."

5. Denial of illness is not uncommon among doctors, but to delay diagnosis and treatment can be deadly.

6. No procedure or remedy is sacred in medical practice. Gospel may become garbage before many years pass.

7. Patients go to quack doctors for many reasons and among them are these factors: A. Inability of standard medical care to bring about recovery, B. Sometimes the high cost of medical care with resultant anger, C. Arrogance of some doctors and the apparent compassion of the quacks.

8. Even if you are helpless in a given medical situation, your presence is often of great comfort and much appreciated.

9. I have learned a great deal from listening to nurses and aides.

10. Be willing to listen to advice-givers even if it means a person lower on the totem pole than you.

11. Successful doctors are: compassionate, intelligent, informed, organized, and possess a reasonable degree of emotional stability.

12. Expect that your hand will be bitten occasionally by the very one you are feeding. Some patients are like that. Gorbachev let the lion out of the cage only to be eaten by it.

13. Happiness is not always gained by making lots of money. It is more apt to be gained by reaching other goals

such as feeling good about your life, an awareness that you have not lived in vain, and having the assurance that you have given back as much or more than you have taken.

14. Much that you hear and read as you pursue your continuing medical education is not very helpful, but occasionally a pearl is dropped which will be of immense value. Don't miss it.

15. It is a sign of your age when you notice that kids are doing open heart surgery.

16. If you are spending more time looking at the nurse than at the monitor, then you have a problem. I would suggest you solve it.

17. The doctor who fathers two babies in eleven months probably flunked his course in contraception.

18. The Salvation Army likely will be on the front row in heaven. Doctors who work more for love than for money I suspect will be too, and maybe even a few psychiatrists as well.

19. It is bad enough to wake up in the hospital, but it is worse to wake up in jail, or not to wake up in the funeral home.

20. Obesity and cigarette smoking are detrimental to our health and longevity for certain. To remedy the situation is virtually impossible for most sufferers.

21. Best way to insure that your patient will improve is to declare to the family that the patient will not live until morning.

22. The cost of medical care is out of control. It is a complex issue. One reason is that most Americans expect to drive a medical Cadillac when all they need is a Ford.

23. It is degrading and sloppy to keep old and torn magazines in the waiting room.

24. I need special help in these decisions: normal delivery or caesarean section, observe longer or go to surgery, admit the patient to the hospital or treat them as an outpatient, advise chemotherapy or let nature take its course, go to the emergency room at 2 a.m. to see the patient, or give advice over the phone, continue life support or stop it.

25. We don't like peer review and we don't like examinations. We don't like to be told what to do. Without this sort of thing, however, some of us would drift into nothing.

26. The country doctor and the aura about him is passing from the scene. I am not sure that what is taking its place will be an improvement.

27. Medical advances in the past 100 years are unbelievable. A hundred years from now we will look back on this day as a day of ignorance I suspect.

28. It is bad enough to have to go to the doctor, but it's worse to go to the funeral home.

29. The doctor who refuses to adequately treat headache victims would benefit from a three-day hemiplegic migraine attack.

30. It doesn't seem right. As a man gets older, his brain shrinks and his prostate grows.

31. We presently keep dead people alive in nursing homes all over the nation. The sooner we are able to change this the better for the sick and suffering who can be helped.

32. A disease becomes reality when we or a member of our family, are afflicted.

33. The doctor who has no time for the emotionally ill would be a better doctor if he had to suffer from an obsessive-compulsive neurosis for six months.

34. The patient who complains about the hospital food when much of the world is hungry, does not evoke my sympathy.

35. There are good and bad doctors, good and bad patients. When the good patient and the good doctor relate, it can be great. When the bad get together it won't be good.

36. Gratitude can be expressed in many ways, not the least of which is the earnest and sincere look in patients' eyes when they, in their own way, say "Thanks for saving my life."

37. If there is a right to life — and there is, then there should be a right to death.

Part Three:

Essays On The Current Social Scene

—1—
Brickbats And Bouquets

(Written in Spring 1992) Run for public office and the bombs start falling when you are fine-tooth combed. The presidential primary elections of 1992 are in progress and who knows better than Governor Bill Clinton about brickbats. He is being nailed to the wall day after day. First, he has been lambasted because of alleged sexual misbehavior. He is now castigated for a letter he wrote in 1969 about his alleged unpatriotic response to military service. And so it has been through the ages. In the intense rivalry, as candidates thrash it out in the public arena, it seems that the strongest candidate emerges often as the one who has collected the least amount of dirt in the mud-slinging process.

And now the scene changes. Death has overtaken one of our fellow politicians and now it is bouquet time. No more brickbats, no more catty remarks, no more probing into the sexual or financial misdemeanors of the departed colleague. Suddenly we start saying all the good things we can in our attempt to white wash the departed and impress if possible the keeper of the pearly gates. Yes, it is bouquet time, big time. I sometimes wonder why we do what we do. Maybe it is this way. During life in the heat of the battle, we throw our bricks. But our adversary can defend himself and clobber the assailant if he is mistaken. In death a poor soul can't defend himself, so we say nice things and give him the benefit of the doubt. Sort of nice. Let's keep it up. Yes, please say nice things at my funeral. Omit the bad stuff and stick with the good. I think we would all like that.

Meetings

I long for the day when committee meetings can be brief, to the point, productive, and at least worth attending. I know deep down that this will never happen so long as mankind has a mouth that speaks volumes and ears that hear little. I dream about it anyway. I saw a sign in an office once that said, "God has promised me that there will be no committee meetings in heaven." If that is true, I'll apply for admission. The skilled chairperson can ease the pain to some degree at these sessions, but no anesthetic in the world would eliminate all of the suffering.

Church board meetings, where peace and tranquility from the sinful world should exist, can sometimes be killers to endure. The fighting in God's name and in his house can get truly disgusting. Then there are the town council meetings where inevitably certain people who love to feud and fight show up and a free-for-all may break out.

Hospital meetings are endless sometimes. Monthly scientific sessions where a big city doc comes out to show slides, for instance, followed by business meetings and arguments seem to go on and on. Then there are the Infection Control Committee, the Utilization Review Committee, the Pharmacy Committee, the Accident Prevention Committee, and how to keep personnel sane committee, who must have their meetings.

Then there is that grand and glorious invention of some government agency that had a nightmare and dreamed up Peer Review. These committees decide if a doctor is good, or bad or indifferent and send him little love letters telling him what they think. They review a medical scenario from the chart only after the event is over. They have the advantage of hindsight which is 20/20. This is an altogether different situation from the struggling and sleepy doctor at 2 in the morning trying to wrestle with a medical problem and do the right thing. He has to keep the patient in mind, keep the relatives happy, the Medicare people pacified, and at the same time he must remember the malpractice attorneys who are circling waiting for the kill. To keep Peer Review quiet and off the doctor's back is no small task. As a matter of fact, it is just about an impossible task on occasion. Are we doctors getting paranoid, nervous, harassed, edgy? You got it right if you say "yes." When the preacher, priest, or rabbi comes by to make a call on the patient for comfort and healing, please let him spend as much energy on the doctor as the patient. Both are presently an endangered species.

Indiana State Medical Society Annual Meeting November 1990

Another meeting! Meetings, meetings, meetings. Will there never be an end to life's obligations? At 67 I look at meetings in a bit different way than I did at 27, believe me! I don't go to so many, I don't get as excited as I used to. I don't get worked up about a lot of things that I used to. Who is it that loves to attend medical meetings anyhow? Well, doctors, of course. But what kind of doctors? Doctors who are politically motivated, doctors who like *old home week*, and doctors who like to get involved in the rough and tumble of organized medicine. I for one, prefer to do other things, such as write, read, wipe snotty noses, and listen to the woes and tragedies of my fellow man. But I am happy and even delighted that there are docs who do what has to be done. Every group of professionals and workers needs to have its concerns made known and its interests protected. That is what is done at these meetings. Preachers, educators, administrators, and workers of every kind have meetings. Policies are made, arguments erupt, business is done, fur flies and eventually the closing session is over.

I'd like to offer these suggestions about meetings: 1. Keep it simple. Speeches can be so erudite that no one knows what is being said. Speeches should consist of simple words, short statements, and be seasoned with a bit of humor. That helps a lot. 2. Don't talk too long and keep it short. 3. Don't keep it entirely objective, throw in some personal things too. That helps a good deal.

And then finally, I suppose that I could wish that organizations could get their work done without spending so much money. When I see the financial statement of the Indiana State Medical Society and the thousands of dollars that are spent on meetings, and realize that there are many people out there who are not getting adequate medical attention, sometimes through no fault of their own, I must say that this does bother me. I am not sure that anything can be done about it, but it still bothers me.

Jargon

I love America. In these days of the crumbling of communism, with all its chaos and confusion, I am especially fond of my country. We excel in the democratic process, we are rich and prosperous, and most Americans enjoy the good life. Many are religious and people of morality and ethical behavior. We have the greatest national park system in the world. We have great athletes. We are good at what we do in many arenas of life. And I suppose we have the best credit in all the world because our national debt is exceeded by no one. It strikes me, at this moment, that likely no nation on earth has ever exceeded us in the use of jargon. It seems to me that in grade school I could read stories easily and the meaning was clear. Like, for instance, Jack and Jill went up the hill to fetch a pail of water. Now I can understand that. But as I advanced up the academic ladder and as I have read mountains of words in the work-a-day world things have changed. Changed? You bet they have! It seems that every discipline of thought is trying to outdo the other in making material complex and hard to understand. Every profession has its own jargon and it seems we do our darndest to make our thoughts complicated. Why on earth is this so? Why do we insist on sounding so intellectual? Why is it in anybody's best interest for smart people to act this way?

Preacher's jargon is there, doctor's jargon is bad too, but lawyer's jargon is ridiculous. I think I could say in one paragraph what an average attorney says on four sheets of paper to get us thoroughly confused. Speakers in our various professions are no better. We simply refuse to make things simple. We seem obsessed with the need to be high sounding and complex. Someone has given the definition of progress as the ability to make the simple complex. If that is the case, we Americans have achieved Olympic gold in the race for erudition and verbal garbage.

Hoods And Scalps

I'm presently driving my son's Mercedes Benz because my Toronado is having an engine transplant. To my shock and disgust I noted shortly after I got accustomed to this vehicle, that the prestigious hood ornament of this grand automobile was gone — ripped off by a hood no doubt. Now it likely dangles from a chain around the neck of this brave and courageous American. I am informed that collecting Mercedes Benz hood ornaments is the *in thing* right now. Lots of brave Americans out there doing their thing. I think I'll not replace it. Too much temptation for our stalwart youth.

This incident got me to thinking about mankind's compulsion to collect things. The Indians delighted in collecting paleface's scalps. Hunters through the centuries have plastered the walls of their domains with trophies from their hunt. I must confess that this sport has never turned me on, whether it is hood ornament collections, scalps, or head-hunting humans or animal.

I can think of a lot better items to collect along life's journey. How about coins, stamps, shells, or arrow heads? Pretty benign stuff. Collecting money, power, or girlfriends can be daunting indeed, if not dangerous. Collecting friends is something to consider for sure. Some folks seem to have a natural talent for this and it is a marvelous venture. Collecting enemies is a natural for others and some are experts at this. Some people have an amazing talent to turn others off. In the hustle and bustle of big city life, many don't collect anybody — friends or enemies. They are too busy doing their *thing* to bother with people.

I hope that at the end of life's game when the whistle blows and the battles are over that I will have a few friends out there. I know I will have some enemies. I know I will have collected some items that I am not proud of. I know I have broken rules, lacked courage, and made some dreadful errors of judgment, but I hope the angel in me has spoken clearer, longer and louder than the demon. I hope until the end of my life I will have a mind that is open and receptive to new ideas and facts. I hope that I can admit that I am wrong when I am, and not be smug when I am right.

You Have Got To Be There

The longer I live the more convinced I am that one can never fully understand anything unless one has experienced it. A celibate priest may have knowledge of marriage and parenting, but not fully, for obvious reasons. A spectator at the Super Bowl may know all about football, but not really, unless he has been battered all over the football field as the player has. To be a doctor is one experience; to be a patient is another. Not much argument about this. It is one thing to read about and observe addiction; it is quite another thing to be addicted.

This last example was obvious this morning as I listened to James George of Project Caress from Bedford, Indiana. He was speaking to an audience in Salem, Indiana. He was articulate, intelligent, neat, and enthusiastic. Here was an ex-convict, an ex-addict, telling us about his involvement in a government support project to deal with teenagers with substance abuse problems. He had been there, he had experienced it all and he was the man for the job. He obviously was giving his job his best. It was more than a job, it was his calling, his life, his passion because he had suffered and because he stood where the addict stood. He had credibility and he was real. He told us about the program of rehabilitation of our youth with conviction and enthusiasm. It was inspiring, it gave us hope.

To escape from reality into addiction is a world-wide phenomenon and as old as history. Why, oh why, do we let ourselves get addicted? There are lots of answers, lots of reasons, books have been written on the subject and the libraries are full. To boil it all down, the real world can be and often is unpleasant, boring, monotonous, cruel, and dangerous. It can be frightening. It can be painful. It can be intolerable for some to endure. To escape is the answer that many seek. The highly competitive society does cause great stress on those who, because of intellectual, social, cultural, or racial problems have a very difficult time making life work for them. They turn to escape patterns of one form or another. Yet, we all know this is no answer; it compounds the problem. It adds misery, crime, imprisonment, and maybe death.

Lucky indeed is the person born with no deformities or disabilities. Lucky is the person who is intelligent. Lucky is the person who was loved and disciplined and had good role models before him. Lucky is the person who is emotionally healthy. These people usually are successful for obvious reasons. Let them be grateful for their blessings and tolerant and compassionate for the person who is deprived.

James George was no doubt saddled with some real problems and he succumbed to addiction and crime. He was able to overcome this terrible plight by his own efforts and the grace of God, as he put it. To have heard his story really made my day. It gives me hope, it gives me encouragement for humanity.

You're Not Dead Until You're Dead

This quote is credited to the well-known and now deceased, Malcolm Forbes. At 70 he departed this world for wherever. Heart attack. He will be remembered by many as a dashing flamboyant millionaire, and his last great party is said to have cost $2 million. I rather like Forbes' piece of wisdom, "You're not dead until you're dead." It says a lot and if we take it seriously it can add a lot to our lives. I have noticed, maybe you have too, that if we are healthy, happy and productive we act and think as if we would live forever. If the sentence of death is placed upon us by a doctor someday, some die right on the spot so to speak. To live each day we are allotted to the fullest is a marvelous gift that some possess but many do not. I wish I could.

We admire those who work hard, are smart, and amass a fortune. America says this is success, no doubt about that.

And I agree, this is indeed a measure of success for certain. But the thing I like best about Forbes is the philosophy of living each day to the fullest and best. That's great. Three cheers for that.

There are a lot of ways to get the attention of people during a lifetime and leave one's name in the historical record. Most of us are just Joe Citizen and figure if we can get through life in our right mind, make our own way, and halfway realize our potential, we can settle for that. That is about par for the course and not too bad. Many have to be carried through life, many have to be locked up through life, and many die young. But down deep I suppose many of us would like to do a little better than halfway realizing our potential. I would like to leave this world and be remembered as someone who tried to help his struggling fellowman when he could. As a compulsive perfectionistic-workaholic person, I would have at one time wanted to leave a legacy of achievement and few mistakes. But as I have gotten older, I now view things a bit differently. Now I have given myself permission to play, to make mistakes, and tell it like I see it even if I lose a friend or two in the process. I finally seem to be learning to take some, as well as give, all the time. I must say I rather like it.

Two Wheels And Four Wheels

I pass the local high school almost every day and see the sights. I see kids in jeans, stone washed and girls with frizzy hair, acting cool. I see some puffing away on cancer sticks — cool. I see the student parking lot filled with cars. Now this one really speaks to me. Wow! Think of it. Much of the third world is concerned primarily with getting something to eat and keeping away starvation. Our world is not the same, oh no. Our concern is a car to ride to school in or a better car to trade the old one in for. When I went to high school we had two wheels and not four. The yard was full of bicycles. Times have changed, of course they have. When my dad was a boy it was a different world too. Change brings good and it brings bad.

And so the question. Is today's world better than dad's world? I wonder. Yes and no is the answer of course. Sixty years ago I was six years old, in first grade. Depression, the great crash of '29 had occurred. We were poor. Fortunes were crumbling. Millionaires became bankrupt. Tycoons became beggars so to speak in a moment. People were in a panic. Some jumped out of windows and others jumped from bridges to their death. Others used the gun to end it all. It was a bad time for the world. There was no welfare and no social security and no nothing. It was root, hog or die.

By the time I was 16 and in high school things were better. People were eating better and life was going on. Nothing fancy though. Stone washed jeans — oh no, we wore hand-me-downs. Cars in the school lot — oh no, only bikes. Cigarettes — there were very few. Pot — never heard of it. Booze — a little here and there.

Today we are rich but we still have the homeless. Today we have the marvels of medical science but sometimes we live too long as a result. Today, as in every day, we live in a hostile, competitive world. Life is a struggle. Victory is sweet. Defeat is ugly, always was and always will be. Friendship and love will never grow old. They are always needed. There is no substitute and nothing is greater.

Roses And Coke

Three-hundred dozen beautiful roses arrived in Salem today from Colombia, South America. They were distributed to Salemites by the Salem Exchange Club members. Some were gifts and some were purchased. A money raiser for the club. Roses are a creation of God, so fragrant, so beautiful, so perfect. They are loved by people, butterflies, bees and, alas, the Japanese beetle. Everything has something working on it, it seems. What a world!

Now, when you think of what comes from Columbia, immediately you think of cocaine and not roses. Roses bring thousands of dollars to the Columbians but cocaine brings billions. We Americans love roses but I am afraid our appetite for cocaine is second to none in the world. It is a blight to our nation and is an unparalleled problem. We struggle to control the situation, but so far we seem to be helpless to stem the drug tide.

The war on drugs is not yet being won. This is no secret, but a massive effort is being made to deal with the situation. I would like to think that a nation, which can put a man on the moon, can bring a gigantic social problem under control. We have made marvelous progress dealing with our health and disease and injury. Technology has made us the number one agricultural nation in the world. Science has given us a standard of living that is phenomenal. We have dealt with our race problem and slowly and surely we make progress. The cold war is thawing, we are learning to cooperate and not just compete ruthlessly. Barriers around the world are coming down in an unprecedented fashion. For all of this we are grateful and our hopes are rising. The good and the bad is within us and all around us. We strive to eliminate the bad and promote the good. Coke and roses. It truly will be a great day for America when we buy only roses from Columbia.

Bedford Blast

Hoosier Hysteria. Basketball fever. Hoosier Dome, Indianapolis. Damon Bailey! Bedford North Lawrence. Indiana State Basketball champions. Forty-one thousand plus people. What a game, what delight for the Bedfordites. It was a wild and woolly game all the way; only three points separated Concord from the champs. Ah, sweet victory and oh what misery is defeat. Sports fans love their idols and Damon Bailey became the idol of idols after the final whistle blew. He is a brilliant and talented player, a student and all-around great guy, too. He was loved, praised and the town of Bedford was his. Damon has a lot of natural talent and he added to this talent hard work, discipline, persistence, and it has brought him the crown of success.

Ah, success, how we love it, strive for it. It makes life worth the living, it spurs us on to new heights and attainment and how bitter is defeat. It can discourage us and cause us to give up. We can with defeat however, refuse to stay down, get up, dust ourselves off and go on. We can keep on trying, suffering defeat one after another, and finally achieve a victory. Then, how sweet it is.

Tidbits For Mom And Dad

1. Infertility is a great disappointment to many a couple, but too many children can pose a heavy burden.

2. When you have one or two children, you may become over-involved in their life and drive them crazy. When you have 15 children, you line them up once a week, call role, and pray together for strength and protection.

3. Children can bring you heaven on earth or drive you to hell and back. Usually it is somewhere in-between.

4. When you manage to get your children out of the nest, you are likely not off the hook. You will be supporting them in every way you can until you collapse and they take care of you.

5. Don't blame your children too vigorously when they screw up. Remember, you gave them their genes and provided much of their teaching and example.

6. On the flip side, your children need to know that they are responsible when given privilege.

7. Don't permit your children to run over you by whatever means it may take. If they do, they may run over the principal.

8. When your children get into trouble, it is probably best to let them suffer. The problem is, will you let them?

9. When your child is king or queen how sweet it is. When they are in jail or in the psychiatric unit, they need your love and support all the more.

10. It's not that easy to be a good parent, and the flip side says it is likewise tough to be a good child.

11. Children are selfish and so are parents, but parents have had longer to mature.

12. Dependent children should appreciate what parents do for them, but often they don't. What parents regard as a favor, the child regards as a right.

13. I suspect that in parent-child relationships, when all is said and done, more is said than done.

14. Sometimes parent-child relationships gets so bad that the door is slammed permanently on the child. Maybe that is necessary, but I doubt it.

15. A dependent parent may be abandoned by the child and maybe it is done with good reason, but I doubt it.

16. Parents must let children run their own life when they are independent. Children would do well to give the parent the same privilege.

17. Children need and deserve the parent's love and approval even when children don't fit the mold. Acceptance of the child, not necessarily of their beliefs, is crucial.

18. Parents are tempted to push their child's troubles under the rug and that is dangerous. They need to face up to trouble and get help whatever that involves.

19. Parents are tempted to push their own troubles under the rug and this is dangerous too. Children may need to apply pressure to get parents to take action.

20. It is wonderful to be respected and dreadful not to be.

21. It is wonderful to be trusted and dreadful not to be.

22. Sometimes we tolerate a disastrous marriage and stick it out regardless of the consequences, but we cannot live with a live bug in our ear until morning.

23. The person who changes his mind too much is rootless and handicapped; the person who never changes his mind can be just as disabled.

24. To have a *wild* child is not easy, but to have one who sits at home and stares into space is far worse.

25. After a crash, I suspect we'd rather face the policeman than our spouse.

26. If every man and woman had good genes and someone who loved them, the prisons would have few inmates.

27. We often don't like authority figures, but without them there would be chaos.

28. There is one thing worse than being too busy and that is not being busy enough. A workaholic creates problems for himself and others, but it beats starvation.

29. In the search for a spouse, it is important to know the family history of organic and mental diseases of the mate. We don't give this the slightest consideration if we fall in love. Nothing else seems to matter.

30. The next best thing to having children is not to have children.

31. There are experiences in life we would like to avoid and one of them is making a will.

32. Christmas letters from friends and relatives can be delightful but they also can be boring. Keep them short, avoid details, and stick to the items of general interest. Don't brag too much. Admit your mistakes, and speak about your agonies as well as your ecstasies.

33. Child abuse is obvious when discipline gives way to cruelty but the child is also abused if he is undisciplined. Yes, alas, there is child abuse, but I suspect there is such a thing as parental abuse too.

34. It's a good thing women can't bear children after menopause. Grandmas just can't be mothers too.

35. Marriage can be heaven or hell but usually neither one.

36. Clothes don't make the man, but they help.

37. When you think about African children darting under the white man's table in Mozambique to retrieve a fallen scrap

of food, you can't feel much sympathy for the well-fed American griping about the preparation of his steak.

38. One of life's most challenging undertakings is to have a successful marriage and rear children who are prepared to live reasonably happy and successful lives. It is perhaps more difficult today in America than it was ever before.

39. Grandparents tend to be mellow while parents often are tense. I wonder why?

40. The man who empties his pocketbook every day is likely to go bankrupt, but the one who never opens it will eventually be lonesome.

41. It is better to see a hungry child than one who won't eat.

42. Children see and accept or reject people as they are. No strings. No prejudice. We adults could learn a lesson.

National Debt, The Cancer Of Our Economy

I am not an economist. I am a doctor. But I am an American and so I'll exercise my right to shoot off my mouth for better or for worse. We all could agree that the national debt has to be curbed. We all, I think, would agree that to do this we have to either spend less, or take in more by taxation, or both. But that is where we end our sanity and begin to engage in irrational if not stupid conduct. The Republicans blame the Democrats and the Democrats blame the Republicans. The executive branch blames the Congress and vice versa. We refuse to elect the official who represents us and allow him to act in the best interest of the nation. We insist that our senators and representatives make our district or state the recipient of all kinds of government grants, and at the same time forbid them to in any way raise our taxes. As I see it, the mess we are in simply reflects our own stupidity and selfishness. We want services but we don't want to pay for them. Let someone else pay is our battle cry. We want our military base to remain and at the same time suggest that the government close up somebody else's military base. I am growing as weary of listening to the rhetoric of politicians as you are. But we make them do what they do. It's not just the politician's fault, it's all of our fault. We all are responsible.

Do I have any remedy for the sickness that is eating our economy like a cancer? Probably not. I find our political health to be in trouble, but we refuse to apply the remedy. It's the same way with our physical health. The fat diabetic with high blood pressure who smokes too much and doesn't exercise refuses to do what he needs to do in order to have good health and prolong his life. He won't stop smoking. He won't quit eating like a hog. He sits in his easy chair and watches television and so he prematurely dies. Likewise, we refuse to deal with our economic crisis, insisting on services but refusing to pay the freight. It just won't work. In dealing with many people who are gravely ill and who do not heed my advice, I sometimes, in my mind's eye just park my ambulance and wait for the crash. I know it is coming. I warn and I plead but nothing happens. And so I suspect it will be that way with our political life. In order to cure the cancer that eats at America's economic life, we have to do several things. The cheaters on government contracts have to stop cheating. The chiselers have to stop chiseling. The congressmen will have to set a better example of personal conduct. We must demand less and we have to be willing to pay for what we get. Simple as that. Will it be done? Not likely! What will happen? I suspect it will be the same thing with our national life like it is with the fat diabetic who refuses to quit smoking and discipline himself. A catastrophe will result. Yes, I am afraid a national disaster will occur and bring us to our knees. I do have some patients who take my advice and heed my warning and improve their health greatly. Wouldn't it be lovely if we Americans would do what we have to do in order to survive economically in this dog-eat-dog competitive world?

Through Hell To Heaven

In early October, 1991, we decided suddenly to get away for a break. Vermont and New Hampshire would be great, we thought. We had seen the wonderful foliage of the Green Mountains of Vermont and the White Mountains of New Hampshire 10 years previously during peak foliage season. We quickly made our plans, got information from a friend who had made the trip before, got our money, got our bags packed and we were on our way to the great northeast.

Indiana Highways are okay but when we got to Ohio trouble started. The interstate system through much of Ohio, Pennsylvania, and New York is in desperate condition. Repairs and delays were endless, and the roads that were open were a disaster. It was a wash-board effect and at high speeds the car pitched around ominously. The speed limit was 55 but no one paid any attention. Eighteen wheelers were everywhere. Bumper to bumper in places. Danger big time. Knowing that some of the truck drivers were fueled by amphetamines and narcotics was not a comforting thought. We saw wrecks. We saw pieces of ripped-off retreaded tires all along the way. We saw dead animal carcasses along the way.

I took the trip because I was stressed out but this was too much. I honestly felt like I'd rather be a passenger in an Indy 500 racer than where I was, but we had no choice but to go and hope and pray.

It became evident to me that our interstate system, in the northeast at least, is shot. We have torn it apart. With too many vehicles, going too fast and carrying too much freight. By the time the roads are resurfaced they are torn up again. The only hope I believe is for public transportation to return to the American scene. Railroads, commuter trains, and air travel has to replace the highway system. Next trip, I will be in the air or else I won't leave town.

Perhaps the highlight of our trip was the Von Trapp Family Lodge in Stowe, Vermont. Last year we had been in the Bavarian Alps of Germany and Austria. The landscape we saw in Vermont was similar to what we had seen in Europe for sure. The Von Trapps chose Stowe, Vermont for the very reason that they felt at home there. The lodge consists of many buildings surrounding the main structure. The architecture was that of German and Austrian alpine villages, picturesque, neat, inviting. During our three days we saw nothing but sheer beauty including many quaint villages and the grand opulence of the George Washington Hotel sitting in its majesty in the valley at the foot of the famous Mt. Washington. We left heaven to return to our southern Indiana home. We had no alternative but to return the same way we came, so once again we braced for the rat race of getting home alive. We saw one bloody wreck and the back-up of traffic was at least five miles in Pennsylvania. Believe me, the next time it will be travel by air and rental car.

Pearl Harbor

I was sitting at my desk on Sunday afternoon on the seventh day of December 1941. I was a freshman at Wheaton College studying my zoology lesson. I switched on the radio and the news was on. Pearl Harbor had been attacked and our fleet and air bases were in ruin. The impossible had happened. The long dreaded war was reality. The news ripped through America and overnight the country was changed, never to be the same. There is no unifying force greater than facing a common enemy. Whereas before Pearl Harbor we were a fragmented people, afterwards we were one. We clenched our fists, quit our bickering, and got to the business at hand.

Students began leaving the campuses in increasing numbers all across America. There were volunteers for the military from every walk of life. The enlisting stations throughout the country could hardly handle the throng. The Navy offered an opportunity for college students preparing for a career in medicine to join their ranks on the premise that we would be allowed to finish our training and go into the Navy as medical officers. I leaped at this offer and was inducted. I finished my freshman and sophomore years at Wheaton and then was sent to a Navy V-12 unit at Tufts College, Boston, Massachusetts and there I finished my premedical training in uniform. After that I spent the summer at Memphis Naval Hospital awaiting the opening of medical school in 1944 in Louisville, Kentucky. To medical school I went and put my sailor suit down for a midshipman's uniform. The war was over at the end of my freshman year. I continued on until graduation as a civilian. In 1950 I went back into the Navy as a medical officer during the Korean conflict and was aboard the Navy ship USS Delta AR9. Pearl Harbor is an example of failure to prepare for an event that one never felt could happen. Even when the Japanese were going into the vertical dive-bombing formation, our military people wondered why on earth our air corps was practicing on Sunday morning. Only when the bombs fell and the explosions and death followed did we realize what tragedy awaited America in that moment. Never had we been more humiliated and soundly beaten than on that fateful Sunday.

Today, Saturday, the 7th of December, 1991, I sit at my desk again. Only this time I am in Salem, Indiana, and I am a gray-headed doctor on third base heading for home. I still am a student; I learn every day. Lots of water has gone under the bridge since Pearl Harbor. I have been reasonably successful and have achieved many of my goals. I have been fortunate. I have been blessed. I came into this world with reasonable equipment to be a productive citizen. I have been lucky. No disasters have cut me short. I look forward to the last lap of the journey with joy and expectation.

Pearl Harbor transformed America from an isolated and untested giant into a powerful military, economic, and political colossus. We are an example to all the world. The world admires us and wants to be like us. They come to us and want to stay. We have our own serious problems, like all the nations have had. Can we survive prosperity? Can we survive our crime, our drug addiction? Can we be the moral force of which we are capable? Will we come together as a nation as we did on December 7, 1941 and face our enemy that would destroy us from within? I suspect that the outcome of this struggle is still uncertain. I suspect that the odds of failure are greater today than they were in December 1941. I suspect that we are our own worst enemy, more than the Japanese. I know that if the sleeping giant of America awakens and answers the call, it can solve the problems, survive and continue to be a light unto the nations of the world.

The Swatted Fly

A big, big fly has been zooming around our room where we are reading. We don't like flies. They bother us. We can do very well without them. The fly swatter was produced and the fly conveniently clung to the wall awaiting his demise. Easy shot. Dead fly. Good job.

Somehow this fly story bothers me some. In some ways it seems unjust that we should eliminate a living creature with so little excuse and reason to do so. And yet, what difference does it make? A fly is of no value or is it? Is this truly injustice? Killing flies is nothing compared to killing cattle, fish and fowl for human consumption. All of nature illustrates the point that survival of the fittest is a fundamental rule of life. The big fish eat the little fish. Polar bears eat seal and the lion eats everybody. From one point of view there is a cruelty to life that is necessary for the ongoing of life on this planet. Everything and everybody has something working on it. The struggle to survive is basic to the existence of life. Without struggle we would not grow and develop. Without the threat of death, life would lose its meaning. Without death there cannot be birth and the continued existence of mankind.

And so little fly, do you matter to anyone? I am sure you do. In the creator's design for the earth, everything has its place, its use, its reason for existence. It is indeed a dog-eat-dog world. That is the way God made it and I don't think of a better way to do it really.

I trust we all can agree that cruelty is unjustified whether it involves flies or humans. I think we all can agree that indiscriminate killing is to be abhorred. I think we all can agree that a goal of mankind should be to live together in cooperation and peace rather than ruthless competition and unnecessary killing. Without question, we have found it is more blessed to give than to receive. Saving a life brings more joy than taking a life and kindness is better than cruelty.

Television

I sat in front of my first TV set in 1948 in the den of Dr. Baker's home. He was on the staff at Waterbury Hospital, Waterbury, Connecticut, and he had invited the interns over for the evening to watch the New York Yankees play the Boston Red Socks. The set was tiny, the screen only 6 inches in diameter and it was round, black and white and a bit snowy, but it was real, real TV! Wonderful TV! Imagine, watching a ballgame going on in New York city 200 miles away? What a thrill! I'll never forget that night.

Forty-three years later I sit in front of my color TV, beautiful big screen and watch the ballgames. No comparison in the reception and the programming. Now we can watch by satellite events around the world. We can even be on the front lines in the battle zone of a real war. We can see king's crowned, riots in progress, and see children starve. We can see police beating criminals and tornadoes reducing the landscape to rubble. We can see flood waters carrying away everything in sight.

We can be educated by television. We can become knowledgeable about the world around us. We are entertained by the television, big time. TV has revolutionized our way of life and its influence on our thinking and behavior is profound.

We cringe at the violence and barnyard morality displayed on television and know beyond a shadow of a doubt that this leads us down the wrong path. But it is like life in general. There is out in the world all manner of opportunity to go forward or to go backwards. It is up to us. We can walk the broad way to destruction or the narrow way to the good life. There are many things that influence our behavior and TV is one of the most powerful. It is up to us to use the facility for good or for evil. It is like so many other things in this life.

My son-in-law spent his last days watching TV. To him it was a God-send. He was bed confined and dying of cancer. Television was his friend and it made his last days bearable.

Chet And Norma

The year was 1944. The place was the anatomy dissection room at the University of Louisville Medical School. The person was Arch Cole, Professor of Anatomy. Dr. Cole came by my dissecting table one day as I was working on my cadaver and said that he would like to speak to me after the session was over. I naturally sensed that something must be wrong and regarded the request with some alarm. At the appointed time, Dr. Cole made an unusual request of his medical student. He asked if I would teach a young couple's Sunday School Class at the Fourth Presbyterian Church in Louisville where he was superintendent of Sunday schools. He was unable to secure a teacher and asked if I would take the class. He knew I was religiously inclined since I was planning to go overseas to do medical missionary work. I agreed to take the class.

For three years I enjoyed my responsibility with this group of couples, some older and a few younger than myself.

In the class was a couple named Chet and Norma Crumbo and I remembered them mainly because Norma was a beautiful girl. She was queen of Audubon Park, the subdivision where I was reared. Chet was a B2 bomber pilot during the war and returned to the States after the war was over. He married Norma and they became involved in the Sunday school class. After three years I gave up the class and moved away to Philadelphia to do my internship.

Forty-five years later I received a letter from Chet Crumbo. He had seen my picture in the Louisville *Courier Journal.* I had been written up because of a book I had published about my journey as a country doctor. It was a delightful letter, warm and friendly, and he seemed ecstatic that he had found a long lost friend. I wrote to him and promised to give him a call. A few weeks ago I called Chet and we had a great time on the phone and we met later for a session of sharing and reminiscing. Recently we had a great time together in Salem. Together we walked to the Washington County Courthouse and looked at the cornerstone. Chet's grandfather's name was inscribed. He was the builder. He opened the first stone quarry in southern Indiana near Salem which is operative to this day. Friendship is a great thing. It is actually one of life's grandest joys.

America, Frontier Town

After a two-week visit to Germany, Austria and Switzerland, I have reached the conclusion that America is indeed like a frontier town compared to Europe. Why do I say this? For a lot of reasons. Europe has a history of 3,000-4,000 years while America has a history of 300-400 years. That tells a lot. Europe is mature. America is in its youth. The culture of Europe has been molded by centuries of events — good times, bad times, war time, and peace time. There have been times of pestilence, destruction, and then rebuilding. Europe has learned about life because of centuries of experience while America is only beginning its journey by comparison. There is a saying that as Europe goes, so goes America. It takes us about 50 years to catch up, however.

In Bavaria, Austria and Switzerland, the farms are small, neat, and every space is utilized. The hay fields are in abundance and the grass is cut and raked into small shocks to dry. It is then gathered into storage areas. The hay fields extend up the mountain sides as terracing permits much hillside and mountainside farming to be done. The farmers live in villages and go to the farmland by vehicles, usually the tractor. The cow barns and the family dwellings are under the same roof and are amazingly clean and neat. The houses of the people are attractive with window-boxes full of flowers everywhere. Churches dot the landscape and characteristically have their attractive bell and clock towers in a conspicuous area. Passenger trains are used much more than in America. They are powered often by electric lines overhead, and diesel-smoke contamination is significantly reduced.

The cities are different from American urban areas in many ways. The streets are often narrow and winding. The architecture is that of yesterday and not of today, although many cities in Germany have been rebuilt from the ground up since World War II. The new structures retain the appearance of the old and restoration has retained the flavor of bygone days. Bicycles are everywhere, and motorcycles, motorbikes and scooters are prevalent. Shops are small and attractive by American standards. Prices are high. The cost of food and living is very high. Taxes are sky high. Social services are greater than in America as a result. It seems that the Europeans have not developed the structures for volume retailing such as K-mart and Wal-mart in America and these keep costs high. Gasoline is $3-4 a gallon.

Yes, Europe is mature and America is adolescent. We are still a frontier nation. Compared to many Europeans, we are undisciplined, unrestrained and we kill each other. We litter the streets and often are disorderly. We Americans want services but we don't want to pay taxes. We want our cake and eat it too. Yet, I would not trade places with anyone and leave my American home and way of life. Even with its immaturity, thank God for America.

Oberammergau Passion Play 1990

The passion play is a drama of the last earthly days of Jesus Christ, from his triumphal entry into Jerusalem until his resurrection from the grave. It includes the story of the prophecy of his life from the Old Testament, his confrontation and rejection of the religious establishment, his conviction of blasphemy, and his brutal treatment and death by the inhumane method of the Romans. Over 600 people participate in the drama. The players, including the leading roles, are all local people who live in the small village of Oberammergau, Germany. Professionals from around the world are not included. The play lasts for six hours with a two-hour break at noon. The stage opens to the skies but the 5,000 people in the audience are protected by a cover.

The bottom line of my experience at Oberammergau is simply this. It was worth the time, money, and effort to make the experience possible. The legend of the origin of the play is widely known, but not to all. The bubonic plague that killed thousands in Europe years ago was raging in the early 1600's. It was approaching the village of Oberammergau and the villagers closed the city gates hoping to keep out the plague. Nevertheless, the plague continued to take its toll and the town began to bury the dead. The churches were filled with the prayers of the believers who promised God that if the plague was controlled, they would present the story of Christ for eternity. And so, for almost 400 years, it has been presented every 10 years.

Pilgrims come from all over the world to witness this event. The spoken word is German but translations are available in all of the languages. The play is presented six days a week for almost six months of the decade year. It is amazing to realize that 5,000 visitors come to this small village each day and can be adequately housed, fed, and shuttled back and forth to the necessary places. Visitors are guests in the homes of the German people in and around Oberammergau, and this experience alone adds much to the Oberammergau saga.

Oberammergau is also a resort for winter sports. Wood carvers in the area produce products in demand around the world. The farmers in the area live in villages rather than on the farm and travel back and forth to their land. The barns and the houses are usually in one unit and are kept immaculately clean. The entire countryside is neat and orderly and flowers are in abundance. German discipline is in evidence everywhere.

Civil War Again By Golly!

May 1989, I have just returned from a trip to Georgia and have updated my knowledge of one of America's bloodiest wars; the *War Between the States*. By all accounts it was a ghastly episode in American history, never to be forgotten. But as I pondered how Americans could kill each other, a half million dead, I came to the stark conclusion that we are at it again. We are at each other's throats. The scene is not Gettysburg, but it is the courtroom. We are not firing cannonballs, but law suits. We are not amputating 30 thousand limbs from injury, but putting each other under intense stress and hating each other. No one was really the winner in the Civil

War, but the winners now, hands down, are the trial lawyers. They love it, they feast on it, things couldn't possibly be any better. The insurance companies enjoy these litigious days because their product is in high demand. "Insure to the teeth" is the war cry of today. Get under the million dollar umbrella. There is a potential lawsuit about anything and anywhere and we are admonished to be fully protected and so we are. Have we Americans gone crazy? We don't dig gold in California, we dig it in the insurance companies' tills. Where the dollar is involved, we lose control. We change our personality. We forget our religion if we had any and we put all and everything aside as we slug it out in *ye old court room.*

As a doctor trying to slowly cut down and enjoy my life after working night and day for 45 years, I have a lingering lawsuit going against me. I feel harrassed and ashamed and at times depressed. The number of malpractice suits are skyrocketing. Malpractice premiums are off the boards. If I were kind and compassionate, I should respond like Jesus and say, "Father, forgive them, they know not what they do." But I don't feel compassionate. I am mad. Who wants to live the life of the average country doctor only to face the firing squad periodically. This very morning I was talking to a young doctor who quit family practice after five years. He had two lawsuits during that time. He told me he simply couldn't get over the emotional trauma of the suit and maybe never would. There simply has to be found a better way to compensate a patient when a doctor, who is a human being, fails to be God, and has made a mistake. If there is not a way found, America may wake up one of these days and will be hard pressed to find the kind of doctor they want. Why? Because doctoring is dangerous. My 45 years of practice have been full of stresses and I know many of my readers likewise have stresses in their occupation. But to have added to our usual stress in the medical world, the ever present threat of the courtroom because you had a bad day or because somebody didn't get a perfect result is simply too much. The stress overload whistle goes off and something bad happens. Ask me, I know. I am confident that the threat of three malpractice suits a couple of years ago coming all at once was the reason for my becoming angry, depressed, and eventually nonfunctional.

Lawsuits are now epidemic. They have swept the country. You name it and somebody has been or will be sued over it. Most certainly people, organizations and corporate bodies must be held accountable in a civilized society. No question about that. But we have to be reasonable. We have to limit judgments. Judges cannot give out multimillion dollar settlements on and on. The medical world has seen and fought epidemic diseases through the years. We have conquered polio, tuberculosis, yellow fever, typhoid, cholera, and a host of other diseases. We are working frantically on AIDS. The medical community has done research and research is intensifying as we struggle to deal with a possible epidemic that may depopulate areas of the earth. The medical community is proud of this record.

But, I want to tell you, the lawsuit epidemic is not being fought by anybody. It is certainly not in the legal profession's best interest to do that. Why? The answer is obvious. They make a living that way. Suppose doctors and medical scientists would say that we could make a killing on treating AIDS victims and therefore not attempt to produce a vaccine to stop a possible epidemic. I don't think that would go over too well in the world community. Well, as physician, I am screaming that there is a lawsuit epidemic sweeping the nation and what do some attorneys do? Instead of fighting the epidemic, they intensify it by advertising on radio, television, and in the newspapers for dissatisfied people to come to them to initiate a lawsuit. That simply throws gasoline on the fire. Am I exaggerating here? Am I painting an unrealistic picture here? Sure, to some degree, but, there is a significant element of truth in what I am trying to say. The bottom line in all of this, of course, is the almighty dollar. We all love the dollar, let's face it. But until and unless we insert some discipline into our personal relations regarding lawsuits, then the civil war will go on and blood will continue to flow.

Sometimes It Works

March 1989, not long after I came to Salem, the drug scene went into high gear in various ways. One of the facets of this outbreak was the delightful activity of robbing doctors offices and carrying off sleeping pills, tranquilizers and narcotics. All of us in those days (15 years ago) had our own supply of drugs in the office. One by one the doctor's offices were broken into and they were relieved of certain kinds of drugs. One doctor even had a confrontation with a wild man one night. He had a narrow escape with his life. At this point, most of us put in alarm systems of various kinds or added other security measures to prevent entry into the office.

I put in a moderately expensive alarm system. Various doors were involved so that if they were opened the alarm would go off. I had sensors placed in the drug areas so that motion would activate these electronic devices. I did not include the windows in the system, that would create too much trouble and expense. The system worked fairly well but occasionally it went off during an electrical storm by accident. I would have to get up and rush over to the office (I lived only 100 yards away) and turn off the alarm. I had an alarm by my bedside so that when the alarm at the office sounded, so did the alarm by my bedside. One night the alarm went off about midnight. I thought of course it was another false alarm, and angrily got up and ran over to the office in my robe and slippers. When I arrived at the scene the bell was ringing and the siren was singing and the dead were being raised, well at least it was loud enough to produce these effects. I surveyed the situation and to my amazement I had walked into the scene of a genuine robbery. I turned off the system and looked around. A window had been broken which was the point of entry. Blood stains were on the tile floor and it was obvious that the intruder had cut himself, but nothing was amiss. John Hart, the minister next door, had seen the would-be robber flying low down Market Street as the alarm sounded. I called the police and they did their thing. Later that night I was called by the sheriff and asked if I would accept a patient from the jail. He was an addict and his behavior was such that they figured he would be a candidate for the hospital rather than the jail. I accepted him and went over to the hospital to check him out. I figured he just might be the one that had broken into my office. I looked at his hands carefully and surely enough a fresh laceration was present in one of his fingers. He denied knowing anything about the robbery but there is no doubt that the doctor who was taking care of him was also the doctor whom he had robbed or at least attempted to. Oh joy, oh delight.

I understand that this man is now rehabilitated. I hope it is true. He could have been my own son. Thank God he was not. I am sure that had he been my son I would have wanted him granted mercy and given every opportunity to get his life in order. From my point of view, I wish he could have been brought to justice and paid for his crimes by doing community work for a year or two.

Which brings up the subject of how society deals with its criminals and offenders in general. The ideal situation, I guess most of us would agree, would be a society which had a justice system that was speedy, fair, and one in which the punishment fitted the crime. Also, a system beyond the reach of the bribe and the payoff. That would be judicial heaven unlikely to be achieved in the annals of history. In the United States we have our share of serious problems with our system, but given the opportunity to make a choice I am quite certain that if I were a criminal or a law abiding citizen, I would rather live in the United States than I would in Iran.

Hamburgers And Hondas

President Bush's trip to Japan in January 1992 brought into clear focus a fact we all had known for a long time. American hamburgers are unrivaled but Hondas are number one in the automobile race. It is difficult for us to admit that despite our military victory over Japan, we are losing the automobile war. We are told that the Japanese have produced the vehicle Americans want, do so very efficiently, and work for less money in order to keep the cost down. Why should this be so? Are we in competition with this superior people and our best efforts will only be surpassed? I doubt that.

It is not unusual for number one to be beaten by the underdog. It is not unusual for the best team to become complacent and get a whipping and this is evident. When we Americans became obsessed with what we can get instead of concern for what we can produce, then trouble, big trouble lies ahead. This tendency is not limited to automobile workers, but has penetrated all of America, so that none of us is excused from judgment. If and when we become more concerned about the quality of our products, the quality of our service we render, and less concerned about what we get, then and only then is there hope for America in the world market.

There is another thought to be expressed. We can live without Hondas but no American can survive very long without the hamburger. When Americans are reduced to poverty and Japanese wallow in their riches, we can't buy Hondas anymore but we can buy hamburgers. Perhaps victory will come at last, when the Japanese are buried in their Hondas that they can't export. Finally, isn't it true that no one will die in a hamburger accident while hundreds will die in Honda accidents?

Snakes I Have Known

Ever since the garden of Eden saga, the snake has been a fascinating and at times a terrifying creature. I have already written about my encounter with the ravages of a rattlesnake bite years ago at Homeplace Hospital. The victim allegedly was drunk when he tried to pet a coiled rattlesnake on a hunting expedition. He was bitten on the hand and eventually was brought to our hospital in the hills in a state of shock. Two weeks later he walked out of the hospital after having endured a near-death experience. I was impressed, to say the least, with the ability of the rattlesnake to make a living for itself.

One day as I was leaving the clinic at Homeplace a man came in carrying a box. He said he would like for me to do a favor for him. I said I would if I could. He asked to go to the lab with his box. My curiosity mounted. He set the box on the lab table, opened it and removed a six-foot rattlesnake; fortunately it was dead. Half way between the head and the tail was a sizeable bulge. "Doc," he said, "I'm a dying to know what is inside that critter. Would you cut him open and find out?" "Sure, I'll do that." Whereupon I got my trusty scalpel and opened up that snake and exposed a nasty sight. It was a partially digested whole squirrel. Much of the hair was gone, some of the bones were exposed, even the teeth. A disgusting and nauseating sight. I went home for dinner. Fried chicken was on the table. I couldn't face it. For a week or more I couldn't even eat meat of any kind. I haven't eaten a squirrel since. I haven't operated on any more snakes either.

The hospital dump was a favorite spot for snakes. We knew that rattlers were to be found, for one had been seen on more than one occasion. Our Dalmation dog often dug and sniffed in the refuse. We knew what was likely to happen and surely enough, one day it did. Our son Rick pulled his dog into our driveway. The dog's face was deformed almost beyond recognition. He had taken a sizable bite on his nose, and his face was swollen big time. I took him to the clinic and gave him three shots of pit viper anti-venom. He lived through it. I was talking to a local resident one day about the snake-bitten dog of mine. He said I should have let him alone. He said snake venom was good for dogs, that they developed resistance by repeated bites. He implied that I had wasted the anti-serum. He made me feel like I was not a very good vet. On the other hand, I am not so sure he was right. He was not a vet or a doc either.

And then I remember Jack, a young man who lived at Thousand Sticks, Kentucky. He went to a church where rattlesnakes were handled in their religious service. He said his daddy handled snakes. He further attested to the fact that the snakes were not pets but were brought in from the wild. They were handled in order to prove that the handler had faith to believe that he would be protected by God. Amazingly, few were bitten. I admired their courage but not their ignorance. The biblical literalist does encounter a few problems.

I have treated scores of snake bites and all but three were copperhead bites, but there is no question that the snake with his venom is no match for man with his gun.

Big Fish Eat Little Fish

Whether on land or in the sea, it is all the same. Big fish eat little fish. It is a cruel world. There is survival of the fittest. Every creature has its predator. Everything has something working on it. Whether it is mosquitos or elephants, gnats or whales that is the case. We are told and believe that all animals except man are on automatic pilot, that is, operate by instinct, whereas man is a rational and thinking creature. Accordingly, we are given the option of cooperation instead of ruthless competition in our relationships.

In the history of the political world, wars and strife have dominated the landscapes with brief periods of peace. In the professional world we see the same scenario. Doctors fight for territory, recognition and for the buck. Attorneys, teachers, engineers, military leaders and all the rest struggle likewise. In the blue collar world, the unions fight management. In the religious world, one religious body fights another for supremacy. Whether the fight is over doctrines, power, or recognition, it's all the same. It is one thing to kill to be number one, but to kill in the name of God is something else. We talk about peace as if we all want it. We hold up cooperation among competing nations or individuals as being the ideal way to go. We know how hard it is to put these things into practice.

I am presently watching the NCAA tourney. For a team to win, it not only requires skill and discipline, but it requires team work and this may require some sacrifice on the part of individual players as well as brilliance and skill. As we all leave the house tomorrow to face our struggle, maybe the victory for the human race would be a bit more secure if we remember that there is no substitution for teamwork. Without it our home, our family, our company, our hospital or our church may not survive.

Have And Don't Have

What we have we take for granted. What we don't have, we want. This observation contains a world of truth I am convinced. It applies to about everything in life. We don't miss something till we lose it. Surely we take our good health for granted. We take our spouses, our children, our position in the community and so many other things for granted. It seems that we can only appreciate something or a relationship if we have at some time suffered loss. The divorced person can really appreciate a loving relationship in a unique way. A good job is wonderful to a person who has pounded the pavements without work. A leukemia victim who has stared death in the face can appreciate life and recovery in a unique way if one has had a cure with chemotherapy and bone marrow transplantation. I can appreciate emotional stability and bask in the delight of normalcy because I have suffered. If we have lost a child, the birth of another has a significance and joy that is special. As a physician I am reminded day after day that my good health makes me a millionaire.

Is it true that what we don't have we want? Sometimes I am sure this is the case. Certainly we want freedom if we are incarcerated one way or another. We want air if we are suffocating. We want food if we are hungry. We crave relationships if we are alone and feel unloved. But there are many things that I don't have and I really don't want. I don't want great wealth, or fame, or recognition beyond my deserts. I do want to be able however to share with fellow travelers. I do want to give and receive. I do want to love and be loved. I do want to help and not hurt. I do want to understand where the other guy is coming from. I want to keep an open mind. I still want to learn. I believe I can and will.

I Wish My Signature Was Worth As Much As Yours

I was signing charts in rapid fire recently at our local nursing home. It was time to write my progress notes and sign orders. Not that I noted much progress with my patients, but I dutifully wrote a statement about each patient's condition. A nurse's aide was watching and made the statement that appears as the title of this article. "I wish my signature was worth as much as yours," she said wistfully. Whereupon I responded that my signature represented eight years of school beyond high school, four years of hospital residency, and 42 years of practice of my profession. And in the process I had worked night and day, had contracted tuberculosis, and had been hospitalized three times for exhaustion and depression. Whereupon she replied that she had only 12 years of education all tolled and was ready for a nervous breakdown herself.

Now this scene reminds me of the fast pace that we Americans insist on traveling. It is go, go, go for many of us. No longer does the average American male come home in the evening to a waiting wife, who has spent the day housekeeping,

A couple celebrating 15 years of marriage may to their friends be a happy and contented unit, but inside the hearts of one or both, there may be hidden despair and frustration. Relationships develop between people which society rejects. But to those who are nevertheless drawn together despite it all, the despised and rejected association brings fulfillment and joy.

Frogs And Racing Cars

I live in a little town near the fair grounds. There is a race track there. On certain nights during the summer I must listen to the sound of midget racing engines doing their thing for several hours. Like a lot of 65-year-old people, I really would rather hear the symphony if I had any choice, but I don't. I can't shut the noise out, I just have to listen. But then I have to realize that there are a lot of people that really enjoy the races and love the noise and the excitement. I am not the only guy in town and what is hard on my ears is music to other folk. Sort of like rock and roll music. My idea of hell is non-stop rock and roll. But at the same time some people think that is heaven. All of this points out the fact that Jack Sprat could eat no fat and his wife could eat no lean. I simply have to remember that our needs are different, our ideas are different, and our appetites are different. It would do all of us a lot of good and promote human relations if we reminded ourselves of this every morning.

Now, I would rather listen at night to frogs out at my lake house. No racing cars, no rock and roll, only frogs and the forest sounds. Now that is my idea of livin' for sure. Teenagers would go bananas on a diet of croaking bull frogs. But the day will come when the appetite changes and the old won't do any more. And so it is with much in life. The fast beat rhythm of youth seeks the fast beat rhythm of the band. The slower beat rhythm of maturity seeks out the calm and the quiet. Only natural. Makes sense.

When people are different and stand out from the rest of the herd, we take notice, often criticize, often joke about it and can be cruel. The serious minded teenager who doesn't party much but studies is often the butt of jokes. It takes guts to do your thing alone. You need a good self-image and a sense of worth to go it alone. Not many can do this or will do this during teenage years.

When the mature person gets out of line it can be hell to pay. To do it differently, to break away from once held convictions, to change one's lifestyle, to change our beliefs, to change political parties, or to engage in different behavior of any kind is to invite trouble. People simply don't tolerate change very well, particularly when they are older. I have in the past year grown a somewhat diminutive beard. The kids and teenagers approve, some heartily. The old folks frown and some even threaten to leave my office if I don't remove it. Amazing how we older folks resist change. When the flood waters come many of the older folk refuse to leave their premises. To grow old often is to stay in the ruts of life and never move a bit. This is not for me. As long as I can keep at the wheel, I intend to change course when indicated. I hope I can speed up or slow down when indicated. I hope I can make a pit stop when needed and then I hope I can get back on the track and give her the gun. I hope I can keep going until I use up my gas and my tires are worn threadbare. At that time I will park it and walk away into the night and keep going until morning comes.

Tidbits For Teachers

1. Democracy is the worst form of government on the face of the earth, except all the rest. Japan educates engineers while America educates lawyers.

2. Make it short and to the point.

3. Make it simple.

4. Smile. It is the shortest distance between strangers.

5. As we are becoming a nation of cities, we gain and we lose. We may increase our income, but we sacrifice our identity in the process.

6. We all would like to think that we are an exception to the rule.

7. We Americans have to win and hate to lose. If we could win all the time life would get sort of monotonous.

8. Glory and achievement may accompany athletic victory, but the price may be high. There is no immediate reward for the book worm, but in the long run, it has its compensations.

9. An examination is like castor oil, we don't like it, but it can be good for you.

10. Every Monday morning during my freshman year in medical school we had an examination in each subject, gross anatomy, microscopic anatomy, and biological chemistry. It ruined the weekend but it prepared us for tomorrow.

11. And a few other suggestions before we declare the Japanese the final victors in the economic war. A. Educate more engineers and fewer lawyers. B. Instant gratification must give way to preparation for long range goals. C. We need more computer operators and fewer rock and roll stars. D. Respect for authority must replace our demand for wild freedoms. E. Worship of the individual's rights need to give way to the rights of society. F. Old fashioned virtues of honesty, integrity, and dependability need to be reinstated. G. We pay the most money to those who entertain us. Perhaps we had better reset our priorities.

12. American democracy provides the people with many advantages, but it can be better. Congress and the executives often are dead-locked and nothing is accomplished. This needs to change. We need a constitutional amendment to outlaw deficit spending by a mandatory balanced budget. A few other things need to be changed too.

13. It's not always true simply because it's in print. Gospel can become garbage in a short space of time.

14. Fifty years ago high schools were surrounded by bicycles, now they are surrounded by sports cars.

15. Fifty years ago we disposed of very little. We slopped the hogs and burned the trash. Now we are replacing things rather than fixing them. When the dumps fill up, what then?

16. Given the same facts, there are many interpretations. It all depends on your bias and where you are coming from.

17. We are presently crying *foul* to the Japanese. We should take education seriously. Instead of worshiping the athlete, we should start paying homage to the scientist.

18. I'd bet on the success of a set of good genes in a marginal environment rather than a marginal set of genes in a good environment.

19. A good school is important in the learning process but there is no substitute for the good student.

20. The best of minds and the best informed clash on many issues. Who has the arrogance to be arrogant?

21. There are times when we are certain we are right only to have to admit later that we were wrong. Some learn in the process and others keep making the same stupid mistakes.

Part Four:

Religious Matters And All That

—1—
God Don't Care A Bit

How many times in your life have you thought this? Many people have thought it and maybe with good reason. At least according to the circumstances in our lives, it would appear that God simply does not care, is absent from the scene, or does not realize what is really happening to us. At times in my earlier years, I wondered and pondered this very question. I think this may be especially true with people who have a religious orientation. There is a prevailing view among Christians that if we are faithful to our religious responsibility, if we obey God as we understand him, if we have been law-abiding citizens, and if we have worked hard and honestly for what we have, then God should reward us in this life in some way or another. The eternal enigma is ever before us. The wicked often prosper and the godly sometimes go through the fires of hell. Five young zealous missionary men went to Ecuador many years ago. They were graduates of my alma mater, Wheaton College. They were all murdered simultaneously by the local people who misunderstood their motives. The lives of good people so often are not spared the horrible cruelties that life can deliver. Innocent Jews went to the gas chamber by the millions and innocent babies die like flies in Ethiopia. An earthquake struck California and the cathedral crumbled, killing scores of worshippers, while the whorehouse across the street experienced no injuries.

As Christians we have been taught that God loves us, that he cares, that the hairs of our head are numbered, etc. Circumstances of life sometimes dictate that this is hogwash. Does he care or doesn't he care?

No one knows for certain the answer to this question and we are ignorant about a lot of other matters as I see it. We see through a glass darkly, to quote the Apostle Paul, but I do think that we know some things. I can understand something about God when I see a family interacting. God thought of families and the idea has come from his mind and actions. Mom and Dad have their children, they love them, care for them, and send them out into the world. They are not puppets on a string and don't want to be. To have their freedom brings with it the possibility of a marvelous life with ecstatic joy. Also, it brings the probability of sorrow, sadness, tragedy, and maybe horror. Our children's joy becomes our joy and our children's pain becomes our pain. I can't help but believe it is this way with God.

Now if we have followed the wisdom of our parents, it may well be to our advantage, but it is no guarantee that we will escape tragedy. So with God. If we have been faithful to our Christian values and precepts, no doubt we will escape many booby traps. Yet it is no guarantee against tragedy. The physical laws of gravity that save us on occasion may kill us when we fall. The immune mechanism of the body that fights off disease may occasionally go haywire and we get lupus erythematosis. Our immune system may someday fail and allow a cancer cell to take root and we succumb eventually to cancer. We are all subject to these laws without exception and without regard to our disposition or personalities.

So, does God care when we hurt? I would like to think that he does. I would like to think that he is our heavenly parent who has given us our freedom but that we are subject to the laws of his universe which are basically put into place for our good.

Some will scream in indignation and say that I am a humanist. Call me what you will. It just seems to me that this makes sense. God made the world. He made us. He thought of families. He cares as Mom and Dad care. He suffers with us and I would like to think, as many through the ages have thought, that we can in some mysterious way communicate with our maker. The scriptures witness to this event. Men and women through the ages have too. Each of us in a sense has to make his or her journey alone. Most of us at some time feel the need for companionship, love, and caring. I believe it is God's plan to have this basic human need met primarily by the companionship of those who walk with us, care for us and hold us when we need to be held. Yes, Jesus talked to God and communed with him as we do, but he also had the 12 disciples whom he loved and whom he needed.

The World Is Hopeless; Let It Go!

This was clearly the message heard from a preacher on Louisville's Christian radio station yesterday. The world is rejoicing because of the upsurge of democracy in Europe and Russia and the Cold War is perhaps the coldest it has ever been. This man of God was not rejoicing. He was angry! Why? Because of his interpretation of Bible prophecy, it was his notion that the resurgence of peace and democracy was nothing but an indication that the end of the world was on its way. Why should this upset him? Evidently, because he felt that President Bush and most Americans and most of the world's population were stupid to think that peace possibilities were reason to rejoice. From his point of view, to seriously talk peace with the communists would only be a step to deception and disaster for the free world. I think this kind of preaching is of the worst sort. It is misguided and does not promote peace. Matter of fact, with this idea, we might as well forget peace and prepare for a war of annihilation. This sort of preaching in the name of Christ and Holy Scripture in my judgment is irresponsible and pokes fun at any head of state or any nation who longs for and strives for peace in this world.

The Devil, Alive And Well

I heard a sermon today about the devil. The preacher was a real pulpiteer. He was an artist at his task. He was knowledgeable, articulate, convincing and interesting. I would rate him an A+ as a communicator. His point was simply that there is a real, alive, active personality, entity, which, if you wish, you may call the Devil. Yes, this was the conviction of the biblical writers, no question. The preacher, being a literalist, regarding scriptures, simply found it necessary to prove his point despite the fact that 20 centuries of knowledge have given us alternative explanations for the existence of evil. The preacher went on to great lengths to insist that the devil, as portrayed by the New Testament writers, is alive and well. Now I'll be the first to admit that it would not be hard to believe in the devil and his imps as we observe human nature at its worst. But this is not the point. I am trying to say that the preacher insisted on blaming the *real devil* for the ills of the world and therefore he is to be fought by spiritual forces of good. Well, let's face it, there is some truth here for sure. Turning the other cheek, returning good for evil, and comforting the broken-hearted. All this is just great, but it doesn't go far enough. You can't cure all disease with aspirin or even penicillin. Life is so much more complex than that. Modern science has revealed the cause and cure for lots of maladies but we have a long way to go. Demons don't cause epilepsy as the Biblical writers thought, a brain dysfunction does. Sins didn't bring on the beggar's blindness in the scripture. Probably congenital syphilis or cataracts did.

In the intense competition that the struggle for existence demands, people are going to get hurt. In the political world as nations interact, there will be bloodshed. The world is essentially a dog eat dog arena and the strong often survive and the weak often perish. Men and women have within them the angel and the demon. Where a spirit of cooperation and brotherhood exist, we can have heaven. Where intense competition and hate exist, hell is the result. No, I don't think it necessary to prove the existence of a personal devil to explain man's predicament. If only we could make as much progress in human relations as we have made in probing space, we just might not have to die to go to heaven.

Christianity And Communism

It has been said that Christianity and communism have something in common, after all both have, in the pure form the possibility of producing a society that could make an abundant life for all. The trouble is, neither way of life is practiced by the people. Strictly speaking then, communism, if really practiced freely and devotedly, could provide a life that is meaningful and satisfying. There would not be the filthy rich and the homeless. The problem, of course, with communism is that it simply does not work. On paper it may look good. In real life, it stinks. The system that was supposed to bring peace and prosperity has in fact brought death and despair to millions of people. We are seeing the drama unfold before our eyes that tells the world in unmistakable language, that communism does not work.

On the other hand, in the western world where capitalism is practiced and where Christianity is the predominant religion, we see glaring problems and inconsistencies. The obvious problems in the USA today are known to all. As we westerners observe the downfall of communism, let us not gloat nor act self-righteous. Unbridled capitalism can and does lead at times to misery and cruelty. Christianity, poorly practiced, can and does lead to self-righteousness, religious snobbery, and has in the past brought death to many in Jesus' name. We Americans have to wince in embarrassment and shame as the world observes our inconsistencies and failures. We have our homeless, millions without medical insurance, the drug traffic, the alcohol agony, our race problems that continue, and our soaring national debt. We seem at times hell-bent to live it up and complain when we can't, and at the same time seemingly be content to let the Third World go.

People of all nations have basic needs, aspirations, and hopes. We are in a sense brothers and sisters in a human family. It will be a wonderful world, perhaps heaven, when we can truly be a world of united nations which have learned to live together in peace and brotherhood. Then we will beat our swords into plowshares and our spears into pruning hooks.

From Bitter To Better

One Sunday night, 51 years ago, I sat in the audience of a capacity gathering in the Wheaton Tabernacle Church. The students at Wheaton College, Wheaton, Illinois, called it the "Tab." The preacher was a student at the college preparing for the ministry. He was cutting his ministerial eye teeth as a student pastor of this congregation. The word was out that this new preacher at the "Tab" was something else. Since Wheaton students were of the evangelical Christian tradition, almost all were to be found in church on Sunday morning and many also on Sunday night. This new preacher's reputation as a thought provoking and spell binding young man of God was rapidly expanding across the campus. I remember sitting midway in the congregation listening intently and watching his every move. He was tall, handsome, and articulate. He held your attention. He was direct, persuasive, and he was a student like the rest of us, but not really. There was a maturity, a style, and a command of his situation and responsibility that set him apart. The open Bible was in his left hand, his right index finger pointing straight at you and his eyes were, as it were, looking straight at you! You were caught up in the drama of his presentation and I am sure many felt as if he was speaking directly to them. I could say he seemed to be a modern embodiment of an ancient Old Testament prophet. He glowed with conviction, urgency, and gave a simple message spoken with clarity and vigor and yet tempered with compassion. His name was Billy Graham.

And now tonight on McNeil Lehrer, fifteen minutes were devoted to a documentary about this intriguing man of God. The story was told of his rise to fame as an evangelist of the conservative Christian tradition. He kicked off his campaign strategy and he held a successful religious crusade in a huge tent in Los Angeles in the late 1940's. Next year he will conduct a great crusade in Moscow, Russia. Wow! What a story! This humble servant of God has walked with the high and low and is at home with both. He has held gigantic crusades in every major city in the United States and is a world traveler. He is a confidant of American presidents and has preached to more people than any Christian preacher has ever done.

Why has he risen to such heights one naturally asks?

1. He has a clear-cut message that people understand and can act on.

2. His charisma is most attractive and he communicates persuasively.

3. He has surrounded himself with talent and his team is superbly organized.

4. He comes across as someone who warns you of evil, upholds a godly life, and yet does so with compassion.

5. He has escaped the tragedy of stepping on a booby trap in life that would ruin it all.

6. He has lovingly embraced all Christian people and has resisted the temptation to exclude or to criticize those who do not agree with him. Consequently, he has a broad base of support in the divided religious community. Protestants of all persuasions, both liberals and conservatives, have stood by him. Catholic Christians too. He shows respect for people and clergyman of the non-Christian tradition. He is positive. He is inclusive. He has torn down fences of race and religion. He has challenged Americans to adopt a lifestyle of Jesus Christ. He has left his mark. He will long be remembered by many who have been shown a way of escape from a bitter life to a better life.

Tidbits For The Clergy

1. Tell it like it is, the truth will be rejected often times. But in the long run it pays to be honest.

2. It is wonderful to be needed and dreadful not to be.

3. When we are up against the wall, we turn to someone we can trust, not the expert we do not know.

4. The clergyman who insists that it is a sin to worry; that depression and exhaustion can be avoided by spiritual resources alone, needs to experience one major depression in his life in order to get his act together.

5. My house is holy and you are not. You can't come in. As I recall, this is about what the Pharisees said to Jesus. My god is better than your god. Forget yours and worship mine. How many of us imply this even if we do not actually say it.

6. Whoever has power is going to use it and that is okay so long as it is used for the general good. This is an ideal seldom achieved.

7. It must be an enhancing experience to be a member of a mega-church. But to have a mega-church we have to have

super stars in the pulpit. There aren't that many out there so most of us must be content with our local situation.

8. So often we are evangelical and enthusiastic about our religion if we think it is the only way to God.

9. In life and death struggles we call our enemies fanatics while we regard ourselves as martyrs.

10. It is more blessed to give than receive until it comes to taxes for services rendered.

11. There are times when we would like to know the future but if we did life would lose its meaning and we'd focus on the suffering that we all have to accept.

12. Stop signs get in our way but without them we have chaos.

13. There are many avenues to success and failure. Your way may not be the other guy's way.

14. There are many roads to God. The one on your road is special but the one on another road is your brother or sister too.

15. Most of us have a tendency to make partial truths the total truth. At 25 we are more apt to do this than we are at 65.

16. Cooperation is better than elimination in the human struggle for existence. But so often conflict is settled by elimination.

17. There is good and bad religion; perhaps there would be improvement if we made our religion relevant and more in touch with reality.

18. Experts abound in the gray areas of life where all the facts are not in.

19. If our next life is no better than this one, would we want to believe in the resurrection?

20. Many religions claim to have a monopoly on truth, but obviously this cannot be the case.

21. It is sometimes beneficial to share your experience with others, but the thing that turns you on may not turn the other guy on.

22. There is a quality in most of us which tells a lot about the human race. When we see an animal or person cut down prematurely, we feel some pain.

23. We work for money and love and both are necessary and rewarding.

24. We purr when given recognition and growl when overlooked.

25. There are many roads to hell and failure. Beware of the one who claims to have all the answers.

26. Today, religion, spirituality, and authority figures are taking a back seat. But guidelines and principles of behavior had better get in the driver's seat or a wreck may happen.

27. There is a tie that binds — love. There is a tie that don't bind — money.

28. I preached a sermon one Sunday in the pastor's absence. During the invitation hymn, one of the older members of the congregation pitched forward in cardiopulmonary arrest. I didn't get asked to preach again for a long time.

29. The Holy Land needs to be officially renamed. Maybe it could be called the unholy land. Perhaps no piece of real estate in the world has been fought over more than the land of Israel.

30. We laugh at the superstitions that govern the life of Third world people, but that probably is not to compare with the disruptions caused by American greed.

31. Give me, oh Lord, direction to deal with my anger, my frustration, and my depression because I experience them all, and so does everyone else.

32. A man's lifestyle often reflects the size of his bank account, but not always. A man's true worth is measured by how he treats the little man.

33. Natural laws we discover, acknowledge and accept. Spiritual laws are less clearly defined and understood. Therefore, it can be a source of unity or division depending on our conviction.

Sabbatical Leave From The First Christian Church

For 65 years I have been found in a Christian church on Sunday except for the occasions when medical, military or travel obligations prevented it. It has been a major influence and motivating force in my life. During these years of exposure to the Christian message and lifestyle, my convictions, my beliefs, and my attitudes have undergone a significant change. Traditionalists and fundamentalists in the church would be apt to say that I have lost my basic faith and beliefs. They might find it difficult to understand why I have changed. They might also feel a distance where there was once a closeness. It seems that brotherhood demands so often that we have similar beliefs, ideals, and lifestyles. I have arrived at a different point of view regarding brotherhood as I have matured. To me, real brotherhood and hope for mankind comes as a result of unconditional acceptance of one another despite our great differences in beliefs, convictions, and lifestyles. For some time I have had an urge to enter into new worship experiences by attending public worship at many Christian Churches, both Catholic and Protestant. I also hoped to include visits with non-Christian religious organizations. Why would one want to do this? Does it mean that I am seeking a new religious experience? No! I firmly believe that hope for humanity involves not only political resolution of conflict but religious, cultural, and social as well. For me to meet and participate in the religious observance of other groups is one way to show them acceptance and respect. I can't imagine that my stance will allow me to accept each and every religious group as equal possessors of truth or effectiveness, but that is not the point. The purpose is to be in a better position to understand the other person's religion and in that way promote peace and brotherhood.

In the pages following I have given an account of my observations and impressions following a Sunday morning visit to several churches in the Louisville, Kentucky area.

Sunday, August 13, 1989
Calvary Episcopal Church

This beautiful cathedral in downtown Louisville with a historical marker out front was the first church to be visited in my new venture. I had actually intended to go to the Unitarian Church next door but found no evidence of any activity and the door was locked. Perhaps they were closed for the summer, so I made my way over to Calvary Church and entered. The cathedral was beautiful indeed and reminded me of an English scene of many years ago. The massive organ, the high stained glass windows, the ornate woodwork, made this a spectacle to behold. The entire service was a new experience for me and a good one. The liturgy, the formality, the kneeling, the words, the expressions were new to me. The communion service was especially meaningful. Called the Eucharist by the Episcopalian, it was served to the people who knelt at the altar rail after going up single file. The sermon was given by a visiting priest from India. The church was by no means full to capacity. Actually, the crowd was rather small. They had three services on Sunday morning and I suppose this affected the attendance at each one. This reflects the falling membership of all the main line churches of today, the reasons of which are many and will be discussed on another occasion.

The Episcopal Church developed from the Church of England as part of the Anglican Communion. There are 11,000 clergymen and 100 dioceses within the United States. The Anglicans of England separated from the pope in the 1500's and formed the Church of England. Anglicans base their religion on the scriptures and tradition, and The Book of Common Prayer is followed. Anglicans are interested in Christian unity. Episcopalians can be divided into the High Church who follow tradition, liberals who emphasize the social gospel, and evangelicals who emphasize personal faith and the authority of scriptures. In recent years there has been a revival of the practice of spiritual healing which requires faith and expectation.

Sunday, August 20, 1989
Evangel Christian Life Center

It was my intention to visit The Church of Christ Scientist today as I drove by the large and imposing First Christian

Science Church in Louisville. A sign out front simply announced testimony meetings on Wednesday evening but nothing about Sunday. The place was abandoned so I went on. I then decided to drive out the interstate and go to the Evangel Christian Life Center, which has received a lot of publicity and is a thriving organization at the present time in south Louisville. This is a live wire and growing church of charismatic tradition. A fairly new campus was evident with an auditorium seating 3,500 people and there were a number of other buildings in evidence too. They included a school and a day care center and I am not sure what else. I entered the auditorium as one service was ending and a second about to begin. I managed to receive the collection plate however in both services. It became obvious to me why charismatic churches are growing. It was like a massive support group in operation. There was music that you could dance to and instruments beating out the rhythm. Handsome men and women were in the choir and on the stage. The songs were rhythmical and the beat appealed to the youth and others for that matter. Folksiness was the order of the day. A number of names were called out during the preliminary services and people were asked to come up front and be recognized for various chores they had (cheerfully) done for the church. A riverboat captain in full uniform came to the platform to advertise a boat ride on the Belle of Louisville. The sermon was delivered by a young and very handsome preacher. He was an excellent speaker and his style was that of folksiness, positivity and certainty. There were no apparently gray areas in his message, everything was black or white. God will do this or do that and God will answer your prayer and will heal you. I got the impression that if the healing did not come then probably it was the fault of the Christian who lacked faith. I didn't see any critically ill people or people in wheelchairs or crutches coming for healing. Nevertheless, the preacher insisted that all Christians can have the power that Jesus had in the first century. At the end of the meeting, groups of people all over the congregation held hands and everyone prayed aloud at once. Some prayed in tongues. I could not understand what was being said, but it didn't matter. Everyone seemed to be happy and in the spirit and some simply were whooping it up. It is heady stuff to believe that you possess the Holy Spirit in a special way above all others. We were encouraged to give lots of money because God would reward us according to our giving. To me the bottom line of all of this is that it does a lot for many people and it is meeting the needs of many people. For someone in the pit of depression who didn't get healed and suffers further guilt, I am afraid such could lead to a worsened situation. It could even lead to suicide. I am sure that what was good for many could be bad for others. Nevertheless, all in all, I considered it a positive experience. They were carrying out the commission of our Lord to minister to the poor and the hungry. They visited the sick in the hospitals and seemed to enjoy that ministry. It is interesting though that if God is able to heal everyone, why should the hospitals contain so many people from their congregation? I am sure that their ministry has kept a lot of people on track, has kept people out of trouble, has lifted the lives of many people to a plane of further enjoyment and I would hope that the charismatic movement is meeting the needs of many people who could not have them met in any other way. Certainly many people are uplifted by a service in quietness and reverence where there is ritual and ceremony. Others seem to need something in between the two extremes. I think it is a little bit like ice cream. Some people like vanilla, some like chocolate, and then some insist on tutti-frutti, but it's all ice cream.

Sunday, October 15, 1989
4th Avenue Methodist Church, Louisville

This congregation is 101 years old and appears to have seen its best days in terms of activity and vigor. A beautiful sanctuary, a massive organ, robed choir overlooking the congregation, stained glass windows; all of this reminded the worshipers about the glory of the congregation in the bygone days. Bygone days? Yes. The huge auditorium with balcony all around contained only a few people. Why? The answer was obvious as one drove through downtown Louisville en route to the church. The years have taken their toll on the entire city. The people who used to belong to 4th Avenue Methodist have moved to the suburbs and the people who replaced them would not be comfortable at 4th Avenue. Furthermore, many other factors in 1989 have affected Louisville's downtown churches. The membership in mainline American protestant churches has been on the decline and this has taken its toll at 4th Avenue. Fundamentalism and the rise of new denominations with a special message have been a competing factor for Methodists. So many forces, movements, organizations compete with churches for the energies of the people. More social and charitable organizations carry out the mission of the church. Ecumenical support groups carry out the mission of the church as well. Medical science, psychiatry, and psychology and other disciplines meet human need which once was the responsibility of priests, pastor and congregations. Authority figures in general have been keenly challenged and this includes the church. People seek and find hope, comfort, love, companionship and strength often in arenas outside the organized church. I have to admit that the church often has been to blame. I am confident that some people do find the crowd at the local bar to be more tolerant, understanding, and loving than so called committed and dedicated Christians.

Will the church survive? Yes, absolutely yes. But it will change. It has to. The eternal truths of the Christian church will survive. Faith, hope, and love will survive. Fellowship, acceptance, support, unconditional love will survive. These elements can be found in many places other than the organized church. They can be found, too, in many people who do not frequent a church but who are carrying out Christ's great commission nonetheless.

Sunday, October 22, 1989
Mount Zion Baptist Church, Louisville, Kentucky

It was a beautiful day in Louisville with all the glorious fall colors. To 33rd and Southern Avenue I went to attend my first worship service in a black church. Mt. Zion Baptist Church was located without difficulty and the building was very nice indeed. The parking lot was full and it had all the appearances of a going organization. Their television program had introduced this congregation to me and I have enjoyed the preaching, the music, and the enthusiasm of the congregation. Two services on Sunday morning were needed to accommodate the people. I introduced myself to one of the men and he showed me where the coffee was and then afterwards took me to the sanctuary. I sat in the middle section halfway down. I was the only white person in the congregation. The service lasted about 90 minutes. The music was great. The choirs were prepared. Instruments there included organ, piano and percussion. The songs were lively and the choir members swayed with the beat. They really sang! The director was a live wire for certain. He literally pulled the music right out of the choir. He sang, he played, he directed. The preaching was by a guest minister. The pastor of the congregation was being honored on the anniversary of his 17th year at Mt. Zion.

I must say that it was a good experience. As a matter of fact, it was a great experience. I was caught up in the spirit of the worshipers and liked what I saw and felt. The congregation can obviously be proud of their church. They belong to a going organization where there is a talented choir and good preaching. The Sunday school was bursting and lots of youth were evident. That church is playing a significant role in the lives of many people in the west end of Louisville.

Sunday, November 5, 1989
Beargrass Christian Church, Louisville, Kentucky

It was my intention to visit the St. Matthew's Christian Science Church today but my plans were changed. I didn't see any activity there. Across Shelbyville Road was the prestigious Beargrass Christian Church. I saw a lot of activity there and so I attended their service. They were in the midst of a million dollar-plus expansion. The church no longer resembled its former appearance. Nevertheless, the place was alive and going strong. Lots of people, all ages. The people were well dressed and represented without doubt the upper middle class. The sanctuary was attractive and very large. There were two choirs and both were talented. Dr. VanNorstrand has been the pastor there for many years. I can understand why. I would give an A rating to the sermon without doubt. The communion was served by the youth. The entire service was exactly one hour and I went away with a good feeling about that congregation. They are doing their job and doing it well indeed.

Sunday, November 19, 1989
Southeast Christian Church, Louisville, Kentucky

I had a never to be forgotten experience on this date in Louisville, Kentucky. Louisville is Baptist country for sure. Baptist Churches dot the landscape and the prestigious southern Baptist Theological Seminary ejects well-trained clergymen into the religious scene year after year. But this church extravaganza was not Baptist. It was a Campbellite gathering of huge proportions. Was it the non-instrumental Church of Christ? No. Disciples of Christ, hardly. It was the Independent Christian Church, aligned with the North American Convention of

Christian Churches. The Cincinnati Bible College and Seminary produces the leadership for these churches. This church complex occupied a huge tract of land on Hike's Lane in the Buechel area of Louisville. It was hard to find a parking place. I made my way to the worship center and the second of three Sunday services was just ending. I entered the library while waiting and gathered information about the church. I found out that the congregation was only 27 years old. It began with a congregation of 50 and now has perhaps 5,000 members. There are three Sunday services in the morning in order to accommodate the huge crowds. Over 3,000 are in attendance during their morning worship services. The facilities are relatively new, functional and comfortable. Everything is on a massive scale. The sanctuary is big, the choir area is huge, and the rostrum is long and wide. The pastor, Bob Russell, is surrounded by an army of 10 associate pastors who keep the huge enterprise going. Support groups for almost every need of mankind are available. Youth activities are in high gear. Sunday school numbers over 1,000.

The service began on the minute and ended on the minute. It was a professional production with lots of talent, planning and coordination. Communion was served expeditiously. The invitation was given at the end of the preaching and many descended to the front of the church and made their way to a side room in order to announce their intentions.

We are talking about a multi-million dollar investment in this church complex. Much money has been given and much money is still owed. Already they are in need of more room. The genius behind the enterprise is obviously to be found in the person of Bob Russell. He is handsome, articulate, prepared, and a pulpiteer par excellence. He holds your attention. He is positive. He is convincing. His message is well-illustrated and his sense of humor shines through. He is warm, loving and has charisma.

One shudders to think what might happen should Bob Russell fade from the scene. He would be a very hard act to follow. The multi-million dollar debt that he might leave would be a formidable problem for any successor.

The success of this church points out several factors. 1. Fundamentalism can and does meet the needs of many people whether it is in the realm of religion, politics or whatever. It certainly is meeting the needs of this massive congregation. Certainty about one's belief system is an invigorating thing for sure. 2. A superstar as a leader can and often does mean the difference between success and failure. 3. Southeast Christian Church meets the needs of people not only in the worship experience but by the availability of support groups to meet a diversity of human need. 4. The youth ministry obviously is going strong as well as the Sunday school program. 5. The people of Southeast have given generously of their time, talent and money and are committed. 6. The leadership has not shrunk from leaping out in faith and the people have followed. 7. Success breeds success and that is demonstrated in so many areas of church activity.

I rejoice in this ministry. As a Disciple of Christ, I would not be nourished and fed Sunday after Sunday in this atmosphere. But that does not inhibit me in any way from tossing roses in their direction. It would be a great thing if all the Campbellites could share their flavor with one another. But alas, we seem to have trouble in doing so. So easy to be close to those who do it like we do it. So hard to share with those who are different. I suspect we will have to wait for heaven to solve this problem.

Sunday, December 3, 1989
First Unitarian (Universalist) Church
Louisville, Kentucky

In downtown Louisville I went this cold Sunday in December to visit for the first time a Unitarian Church. The church building was virtually destroyed by fire a few years before and has been restored. The finished product was an amazing structure. The stone walls that withstood the flames were incorporated into the new structure in a unique and beautiful way. The building, beautifully rebuilt, was functional and modern and yet contained the flavor of the old. I couldn't help thinking about that as I sat in the chair awaiting the beginning of services. As institutions evolve, as people change, as structures restructure, as the old gives way to the new, we go through the process of updating and reaching out to the new while holding onto that which does not change. This illustrates a process in life that is played and replayed over and over. For anything to survive in this complicated world, changes and adjustments are inevitable. We preserve what is enduring as we modify, switch, and eliminate that which must undergo a transformation.

I must confess that Pentecostals and Unitarians are not quite the same in the way that they view God, Jesus, the Bible, and other religions. As a matter of fact, they are poles apart but they have similarities too. In both churches are to be found people with needs to be met. If they have none, they wouldn't be out there seeking on Sunday morning. People reach out to find God, to find what is real, to find answers, to find comfort, strength, peace, and serenity. People need each other and need acceptance, need love, need understanding. Whether Pentecostals or Unitarians, they are people who are seeking and who have needs. The Pentecostal Church service meets the needs of its people and the Unitarian approach meets the needs of its flock. I am not the one to sit in judgment and say one is right and the other is wrong.

The service at First Unitarian was an hour in length. There was singing, recitation of liturgy, and readings from various sources of inspiration and wisdom. It was obvious that they did not consider the Bible to contain all of the world's religious truth. There was the sermon and a candlelighting service to express the idea that lighting a candle was better than cursing the darkness. After the service was over, there was a time of fellowship and coffee. I moved on, time was a factor as usual.

How did I receive this, my first Unitarian worship experience? Was I uplifted? Was I spiritually fed? Did I sense the divine spirit? My first answer is that I felt good about the experience because I was entering into a new community of the human family and was being a part of them for a brief moment. That was the best part of the experience for me. Also, I learned from them. It was informative. I enlarged my horizon and took in more of the world of religious thought and expression. The point is not whether I was in agreement with them. The bottom line was that I became a part of them for a short moment and shared a common worship experience on their territory. To me, if there are any answers to this world's problems, whether they be global, national, or individual, it will come through efforts to gain community and to share with and accept those who are different.

Sunday, February 11, 1990
St. Paul's United Methodist Church

This is the church where my friend and colleague, Dr. David Stewart, was an active member. It is where he worshiped for the many years he worked and lived in Louisville, Kentucky. It is here that he was teacher of the Covenant Sunday school class. I decided that I wanted to visit the scene of his church family. The church is located at Douglas Blvd. and Bardstown Road in Louisville. The sanctuary is beautiful and the congregation large. I had the privilege of meeting members of his Sunday school class and had an opportunity to speak to them about David for a few minutes. It was indeed a special time. Martha, David's wife, was in Kenya, Africa at the time.

The service began with a full house and lasted the usual hour. The sermon was good but the hymns were unfamiliar to me. Of course, communion was not served, contrary to the custom in the Disciple's Churches. The choir sang during the collection. The service was well-organized and I was impressed that here was an alive church with an active and vigorous ministry. Perhaps the thing that impressed me most was a project that was announced to the congregation. The church was participating in a program in which volunteers would agree to work for six months with a youth offender. These teenagers had been convicted of a minor crime and they were assigned community projects as part of the program of restitution and rehabilitation. The Chairman of the Committee was asking for persons in the church family to participate. This to me would be a great opportunity to put Christianity into action in a positive way. I hope the church succeeds in this endeavor. I think it has great potential and it won't be easy. There are no guarantees of success. The church has not had much experience in this sort of thing. I wonder if the volunteers will be given instruction and guidelines? The experience of other churches, if any, would be helpful.

Sunday, February 18, 1990
Douglas Boulevard Christian Church

This church is reputed to be one of the more prestigious Disciples of Christ Churches in the Kentuckiana Disciples Association. My visit on this occasion confirmed the church's reputation. The building and grounds were beautifully kept up and the church's location ideal. I asked a gentleman about a Sunday school class and I followed him to his. The class was composed of adults my age, well attended, and taught by three persons. The sanctuary was striking in its beauty. The service moved along professionally and the choir was well trained. The sermon was about divorce, an extremely tough assignment for the minister. No doubt many divorced persons were in the audience that Sunday. He handled the subject with knowledge and expertise. I felt he was able to uphold the scriptures and the position of Jesus, and yet with grace and understanding he took a nonjudgmental stance. In this modern age, many couples are facing the dilemma posed by difficulties of maintaining marriage vows for reasons with which we are well acquainted. He surely upheld the ideal of Jesus in which he made it clear that marriage should be for life and what God has joined together let not man put asunder, as the marriage vows state. However, he recognized that in this day and age the ideal could not always be met and that Jesus, if he were living today, would regard people with compassion and understanding should they come to him with an impossible dilemma of maintaining a marriage.

A couple responded to the invitation at the end of the service to accept Discipleship and asked for membership in the Douglas Blvd. Christian Church. I left with a good feeling. A coffee-and-cookie time followed in the fellowship hall where I met a few members of the congregation and enjoyed a brief social contact.

Sunday, March 4, 1990
Church Of Jesus Christ Of Latter Day Saints

I awakened on this Sunday to a beautiful day. It would be a good day to go to the city and visit another church and continue my project of getting to know new congregations of Christians. To learn to know about a church different from your own, you need to be with them. I think you can learn a lot more from three hours in a congregation than reading about the situation for three days. I went to the Church of Jesus Christ of Latter Day Saints in New Albany. This was the church where my friend and colleague, Dr. Charles Carty, lay in state for his funeral service. The church was located on Slate Run Road in New Albany. The structure was fairly new and provided an excellent facility. There were three services.

The first was a gathering of the entire church in the sanctuary. Here I listened to brief testimonies from members of the church, both youth and adult. They were telling their story, experience and their remarks centered about the theme of appreciation and thanksgiving for the church's nurture in their individual lives. I knew most of the songs they sang and participated. After this service ended, I attended a class taught by a knowledgeable and gifted young man. He used the Bible, the Book of Mormon, and the study guide provided by the church in Salt Lake City. It was a lecture and was well presented. There was minimal discussion. After this the men gathered in one area and the women gathered in another. The meeting was more like a Sunday school class again. It was called a meeting of the priests of the church.

I was well received and the people were friendly. I let one Elder know that I was not a candidate for conversion but simply was interested in knowing more about the members of the Church of Jesus Christ of Latter Day Saints. I admire them for their zeal, commitment, and the good piece of work they are doing for their constituency. Many people seem to need and even thrive on the authoritarian emphasis of Latter Day Saints. Things tended to be black and white and there are no grays. They are unified. They believe the same things. There is no room for theological debate. Women assume the traditional roles of women of many years ago. They take pride in staying at home with their family and doing the things that are obviously praiseworthy. Men are in a position of leadership and women have their clearly-defined supportive roles. The church is rapidly growing worldwide and it is easy to see why. They have zeal, commitment, and enthusiasm. They are aggressive and send out missionaries to promote Christianity. Their program meets the needs of many and is designed to promote and stabilize family life. They challenge their people to sacrifice and put the church first. It is obvious to me that LDS people are doing an outstanding job in promoting their understanding of Christianity. Hats off to the Mormons.

Sunday, March 11, 1990
Graceland Baptist Church

On this lovely warm spring Sunday, I went to New Albany to visit another mega-church. Graceland Baptist is relatively new on the religious scene but in a short time has had fabulous success. It is known for the Living Christmas Tree, the fantastic outdoor Christmas lighting, its 5,000 members, their school and preschool, and now the embryonic university. Obviously, all of this indicates success and glory. Along with it there is hard work, dedication, commitment and sacrifice on the part of many.

The church is located just off Charlestown Road near I-265 interchange. The campus is spacious and beautiful. The buildings are fairly new and functional. The trappings of success are obvious as one drives into the filled parking area and looks around. I entered the sanctuary and picked up several pieces of literature in the vestibule. I was extended a friendly greeting. I was a bit early for Sunday school and the first of two worship services was just ending. I had time to go through the handouts and get an idea of the activities at Graceland. It was obvious that plenty was going on and that this congregation fulfilled the criteria for a mega-church.

At this point I was ushered to the men's Sunday school class taught by one of the assistant pastors. It was lecture style. The lecture was from the book of Judges. It had to do with the covenant between God and the children of Israel. They were unfaithful and so were punished. That was applied to the church today, certainly a lot of truth here, and many in the class approved of what was being said. How did I know? The teacher was encouraged by repeated *amens* from the audience. The teacher came down hard on the church today and the lack of commitment, vitality and concern for the *lost*. He seemed to enjoy what he was doing. It strikes me that some clergymen rather enjoy preaching about the wrath of God.

After Sunday school, I proceeded to the sanctuary and the crowd was gathering. The gathered folk were singing choruses and a handsome young man was directing. People were obviously having a good time as the auditorium filled. The singing stopped and the service began. A long time was taken for announcements and the church seemed to be going in every direction doing about everything for almost everybody. The choir area was filled and an orchestra assembled. The congregational singing was accompanied by the instruments and the percussion and beat was obvious. Tambourines were sprinkled here and there among the choir members and the music was lively, rhythmical and people in the audience were really getting into it. Some were keeping time with their bodies, others held their hands high and it became clear that this was no typical Southern Baptist Church. Here was a Baptist-Pentecostal gathering and this had to be a first for me. There followed a period of praise and thanksgiving and the people really got with it at this point and were having a good time.

The sermon was 45 minutes in length. The preacher was well prepared, gave a good sermon and was obviously well qualified to lead a mega-church. He was able to exhort the brethren to more commitment in evangelism and I imagine put several on a guilt trip for their laziness. He portrayed a world en route to hell (fire and brimstone kind) unless they heard the message, confessed their sins and came into the church.

I have a hard time with this. To condemn a Moslem to hell because he had no chance to become a Christian is unjust by anyone's standards in my judgment. Furthermore, I have a real hard time with another thing. These people were happy and they were rejoicing in the church and in their Christian experience while all the time knowing that most of mankind would spend eternity in hell. If I really believed this doctrine, in no way could I rejoice and be happy. I would be exceedingly depressed. To realize that most of the Third World already live a hell of a life by American standards and then to commit most of them to spend eternity in hell is just too much for me to accept. A God who would allow a world like this to exist would, in my opinion, be cruel.

The service ended with an invitation for folk to respond to the sermon and come to the front of the sanctuary at the altar rail. Several did and they were met by deacons who received their concerns. On the positive side of the ledger, this church is successful in what it intends to do. It provides a fellowship for many which is rewarding and empowering. It's always nice to be a part of a winning team and a dynamic organization. I am sure the church provides an environment for the development among the people of morality, security, and many Christian virtues. It provides purpose and direction to the lives of many people. It is an empowering thing to believe as they do. Perhaps the greatest weakness of a fellowship of this kind of the judgmental stance that so often is second nature to those who are the most committed. Whenever you are convinced that you have all or most of the truth, it naturally follows that the rest of the world needs to see it as you do.

Sunday, April 1, 1990
Kingdom Hall Jehovah's Witnesses, Salem, Indiana

On this day I did something that I have never done before and I had a ball. I attended the services of Salem's Kingdom Hall of Jehovah's Witnesses. It was a beautiful day, the parking lot was full, and so was the building. There were 150 people in attendance. I knew many faces, many were patients of mine. The building is fairly new and modern, and it was simply constructed and decorated. A large painting was obvious up front depicting the waters of baptism.

A district representative was there. He gave a sound and slide presentation of Jehovah's Witness activity last August in Poland. Three massive conventions were held in Poland with participants coming from many countries of the world. Big time! Sixty thousand people at one outdoor stadium. Seventeen languages were spoken. All believed the same and fellowship was sweet and comforting. The slide show was a professional production and the message was (expertly) communicated. Following this, the Watch Tower lesson was given and the audience participated. Questions were asked about the lesson, and the audience answered as individual members were given the portable microphone. All Jehovah's Witnesses receive the same lesson world over and there is no disagreement or argument over doctrine or procedure. It is a tightly-controlled organization giving no room for individual opinion or variation on matters of theology or church policy. Following the lesson, the visiting district representative gave a sermon which I would rate very high indeed. It was practical, Christian and well delivered.

The songs were new to me. Communion was not served and there was no offering taken. There was a spirit of brotherhood and fellowship. There was conviction, certainty and enthusiasm. Jehovah's Witnesses are growing fast. It is easy for me to see why. They give the impression that Jehovah's Witnesses are very special in God's (Jehovah's) world and to put it bluntly, I believe they feel that they are on the front row of the Christian religions. They believe that they have the true message and that others need it because the end of the world is near. There is an element of urgency. Evangelistic zeal is obvious. Commitment to their task is there. They fully believe the world's ship is sinking and that they are manning the lifeboats. They see that as their primary objective. Energy expended for the sake of making the world a better place to live to them is only expended in terms of evangelism. They would have little concern for the United Nations, world peace movements or other social efforts to preserve the world order.

Witnesses are found all over the world and have been around for over a century. They have an appeal that is irresistible to many. As I see it, they regard themselves as Jehovah's special people having all or most of the truth. This certainly can build self-esteem within people who are fully committed to their movement. There is a fellowship among the members that is strengthening. They do not have complacency, apathy, and spiritual lukewarmness to contend with. There is no clergy. All members are ministers, in a sense, and the responsibility rests on their shoulders. One has to admire many things about Jehovah's Witnesses. The very thing that gives them their zeal, however, tends to separate them from other Christians and so perpetuates the divided Christian religion. There is indeed a fence around Jehovah's Witnesses. People are free to enter but not to leave in terms of communication with other Christian religious groups.

Sunday, April 8, 1990
St. Bertrand's Catholic Church
Louisville, Kentucky

On this beautiful Palm Sunday, I went to Louisville for two missions. One of my good friends and patients was in Audubon Hospital in recovery from open heart surgery. He was reported in critical condition. He had his surgery while a major heart attack was in progress. It was the intention of the doctors to head off the attack but they failed to get there in time. Thus he was suffering the effects of the heart attack along with the trauma of open heart surgery. I went to the open heart intensive care unit and for a moment saw him and embraced his wife and son and made a speedy retreat. The marvels of medical science are here, but the monster of disease often beats us. Anyhow, Audubon Hospital is located near my boyhood home in Louisville. Fifty-five years ago the entire area where the hospital was located had been a woods with a creek and trails. Now a thriving residential and commercial area is in existence.

A short distance from the hospital was the parish Church of St. Agnes and I made my way there for worship. I arrived in the midst of a mass and the church was packed since it was Palm Sunday. I proceeded then to St. Bertrand's Catholic

Church at Sixth and St. Catherine and got a rear seat for the mass. I couldn't hear very well but got enough to participate. It is a beautiful church, very old, and kept up in all its resplendent glory. Most of the seats were occupied by the faithful and perhaps by some not so faithful. I suspect Catholic churches are like Protestant churches inasmuch as bigger crowds are found at Palm Sunday and Easter.

It never ceases to amaze me how Christians worship in such different ways. The extremely demonstrative Pentecostals at one end of the scale and the highly ritualistic Catholic masses on the other end reveal the differences in Christian worship. And then there are all the ones in between. So often, each one feels that his way is the best way; is God's way. I am afraid we tend to confuse the issue by saying "God's way" when we should be saying "our way." The factors that determine how we worship depend on many things. Often we follow the tradition of our home, our parents, and our culture. Then our own individual needs come into the picture. There is our lifestyle, and the segment of society from which we come, which helps determine our church preference. Some like and need rigidity and others need freedom. Some need black and white religion, so to speak, and others are comfortable in an atmosphere of grays. But I believe the bottom line for all of us is to find a place to worship where we feel accepted and loved and cared for.

Monday, May 14, 1990
Faith Christian Center Revival Crusade

On a cool May evening at 7 o'clock we gathered on the edge of Salem for this joint effort of several Washington County churches. Faith Christian Center is a rapidly growing church, fundamental, with a charismatic flavor. It is another example of a phenomenon which is happening all over the

Christian world, namely a resurgence of enthusiasm and participation in a church where gray is rare and where black and white are obvious. And I, of course, refer to the kind of religion that tends to be absolute, authoritative and dictatorial. If one truly believes that his convictions are correct and that those who think differently need to be corrected, it can be invigorating and attractive. The church here in Salem is a new church and is obviously meeting the needs of many families and is growing steadily while Salem's mainline churches are down and are slowly shrinking in numbers. This is a national happening and perhaps world wide in the Christian community. Perhaps this can be said of many religions in addition to Christianity. The Moslem and the Jewish fundamentalist seem to be in the forefront and gathering steam as well. Nothing wrong with enthusiasm. Nothing wrong with people of conviction and commitment. Nothing wrong with growth of that which is good for people and good for the world. The problem, as I see it, is the lack of respect for the opinions of those who disagree that I see among both fundamentalists and, at times, liberals. Often, the liberal looks down his intellectual nose at what he regards as the uneducated and closed-mindedness of the fundamentalist.

To get back to the meeting, the revival team was from Michigan. It was composed of young couples and their families, about 25 in number. They travel about in mobile homes from city to city. These people are talented. The preacher is well prepared and able, and the two hour event was produced in a professional way. As is so often found in these revival events, it is delivered to the people from a lofty height. That is, the preacher and the team are speaking from a position of spiritual heights and authority to a group of people who are down on a lower level of spirituality. The idea is to convince those who are lukewarm or halfhearted to move on to a greater level of commitment. Nothing really is wrong with this. The danger lies in the fact that some can be hurt in the process. The person who is in considerable personal and emotional distress, looking for guidance and help, can, I believe, be unable to cope with the preacher's demands and thus might go out more confused and guilty than ever. The Christian fundamentalist's approach to solving personal problems and giving peace, purpose and power to life is certainly one option for people to take a close look at. Many have found that experience leading to a more rewarding life. But it is not the only way as I see it. There are others. There are more ways to God than one. More than one way to a meaningful, productive and purposeful life. All of us, I believe, need to recognize this, if we are to achieve a greater spirit of community and brotherhood in our search for the good life.

Sunday, May 20, 1990
Crescent Hill Baptist Church

On this beautiful day I visited the prestigious Crescent Hill Baptist Church which has through the years maintained a special relationship with Southern Baptist Theological Seminary. It simply came into being by virtue of its proximity to the seminary, I presume. In my mind I have associated this church with seminary students, faculty from the seminary, outstanding ministers who have been pulpiteers par excellence, and possessing unusual qualities of leadership. This was my first time to enter this church and it was indeed an event I shall long remember. Located in a well-kept neighborhood of Crescent Hill, the buildings and grounds of the church are lovely and more than adequate. I asked for help in finding a Sunday school class and was ushered into the *Fishers Class*, a small group of adult men. A lively discussion and an able leader was in evidence. As I had hoped, the conversation touched on the issue of the Southern Baptist Theological Seminary and their controversy. Crescent Hill would, of course, be aligned with the moderates rather than the fundamentalists who are determined to clean out heresy which they regard has infiltrated the seminaries, Southern in particular.

I made my way to the sanctuary which was comfortably filled with many in the balcony. The service was different, I mean really different. I have been a deacon and a Sunday school teacher in Southern Baptist Churches for many years in the past and I have heard many sermons from Southern Baptist ministers. This service was the most unbaptistic service I have ever witnessed. Frankly, I loved it. I rejoiced in it. I felt God's presence anew. Outstanding were two events in the service. One was a dance of four people accompanying the singing of *Amazing Grace*. Sounds really far out, when actually it was a very special and lovely experience for all of us. Then came the sermon. Dr. Shoemaker is a handsome and articulate man speaking with a southern accent. He exudes warmth and conviction. His sermon was on sorrow and joy, stories and songs. He sat down with his cello in his arms. He is an accomplished musician. He told of his experience with his emotions of sorrow and turbulence that has recently occurred in his life. He spoke of being able to express himself with the help of his cello and he played bits and pieces of some of the wonderful and majestic songs of faith. Sandwiched between songs, he told stories to bring out his message. He got the message through. I suspect he is a superstar at what he does although I have heard him speak only once. The service was over. I was greeted. I felt good, so good about this experience. If the fundamentalists of the convention consider this kind of Baptist worship and flavor to be objectionable and to be discarded, then I say a tragedy is in the making. In trying to clean out the attic of undesirable junk, the convention will toss out a diamond. If Crescent Hill and what it stands for is on their hit list, they will indeed throw out the baby with the bath water.

Sunday, July 8, 1990
Shawnee Christian Church

A very hot day it was, but the cool comfort of the church house was a welcome relief. Relocated in the Shively community of Louisville, this church once occupied a building on Broadway in the Shawnee Park neighborhood. The move came about 25 years ago when the Black population of Louisville occupied the west end of the city. As many white families sold out and moved, so did many clubs, organizations and churches. The facts of life bring this about despite the fact that in an ideal world the attitude of acceptance should prevent this from happening. The church at the time was thriving and had 800 members. It had good leadership and was meeting the needs of many people. Alas, the move proved to be the beginning of a series of misfortunes that resulted in the current membership of perhaps 100 or less. Their present attendance averages 50-70. At the same time this was occurring, the mega-church, Southeast Christian in Louisville, was growing from a group of 50 and has now resulted in a congregation of 5,000. This event is representative of a phenomenon that is occurring in many neighborhoods in the USA. In part it can be explained by the fact that churches, like stores, restaurants, service people, and all who are out there in life's competitive race will have periods of success or failure. There will be periods of growth and expansion and at times shrinkage and death.

Shawnee's experience represents a development in mainline Protestant churches that is occurring throughout the USA. Many mainline churches such as United Methodist, Episcopalian, Presbyterian, American Baptist, and the Christian Church (Disciples of Christ) are in a period of recession and loss of membership and strength. The reasons are many. Mainline churches have traditionally been downtown city churches. With the population shift these churches have seen a loss of membership. Additionally, liberal Christianity has invaded the mainline seminaries and institutions and this has brought about an emphasis on ecumenical activities, and an acceptance of *saving the world* rather than saving souls. Mainline churches have tended to think more in terms of human rights, minority rights, and social justice. Their idealism has brought into the forefront the emphasis on promoting world brotherhood, rather than beating drums for America in every international situation. They have tended to see the Christian Church as perhaps the best way to God but not the only way. They have looked on other religions as opportunities for discussion and brotherhood rather than as objects to be eliminated by conversion to the Christian faith in the American style. The result of all this has tended to produce a malaise that is pervasive in many churches. On the other hand, the churches that are growing and currently popular in the American scene are those who we regard as fundamental and have a more dedicated evangelistic fervor than mainline churches. Southern Baptist, especially at this time, demonstrates this. The fundamentalists have won the struggle with the liberals and are cleaning house at this very moment in history. Mormons, with their exclusiveness, and their militant evangelism are growing. Pentecostals are growing. The churches where religion is black and white without grays are popular today. The religious groups that emphasize patriotism, America first, and individual soul saving and spiritual advancement are growing. Indeed it is energizing and flattering to think that one's religious group has all or most of the truth.

As I see it, the Christian message has penetrated much of American culture and the church's job is often being done in many arenas, but not in the name of the church necessarily. Since the days of Christ, the world has never been the same. People are regarded in a new light. They are important. We see the church's message being carried out all about us. The work of hospitals, health care deliverers, mental health people, social workers, charitable organizations by the hundreds, demonstrate this effectively.

As a member of a mainline church, the Christian Church (Disciples of Christ), I am a member of a shrinking group. If Americans get their spiritual needs met in a fundamentalist atmosphere, I have no quibble. I could wish the fundamentalists would grant the liberals the same courtesy. I wish the Mormons would evangelize the unchurched primarily, rather than trying so hard to convince members of other churches to become Mormons. Probably the liberals among the Southern Baptist need to find another home. I don't think they can feel at home with a Southern Baptist convention any longer. When one is looked upon as a rebel, as a traitor, as a second class citizen, there needs to be a divorce. Inevitably, Southern Baptists will have to go through the final agony of this separation. I suppose all of this represents a universal inclination of mankind to look after his own self-interest, to consider his own religion the best, and to think of himself as the center of the universe and to believe that his world view is correct.

Back to Shawnee Christian Church. A series of misfortunes in leadership, along with the phenomenon as explained above, have reduced the church to a fraction of its former membership. Nevertheless, it was a delightful Sunday as my wife and I visited and worshiped. The pastor, brother of my wife, gave an interesting and thought-provoking message and it was well done, very well done. The entire service was appreciated. A fellowship meal followed in a beautifully occupied area made for that purpose. The people at Shawnee have a *Roll's Royce.* I hope it can be put to even greater use for the benefit of others in the days that lie ahead.

Tidbits For The Clergy

1. There is satisfaction in being a servant of the people, but it can have its downside.
2. The clergyman sees people when they are good, the lawyer when they are bad, and the doctor sees them as they are.
3. Discipline is like castor oil. It tastes awful but it is good for you.
4. Christmas can be glorious or painful depending on your circumstance.
5. Flood waters wash away all in its path, churches, saloons, and brothels. Regardless of our credentials, we are all subject to nature's laws.
6. Freedom is an American heritage, but unless it is accompanied by discipline it can take us down the road to despair and an early grave.

7. There are some in the world about whom you can say, "to know them is to love them." Usually it turns out that they are loving people.

8. The homophobic person would likely not be one if he had a child who had a gender orientation problem.

9. Christmas is the grandest time of the year if you can live through it.

10. The faith healer who says doctors are unnecessary would learn a much needed lesson by having a kidney stone attack at 2 a.m. May he have one soon.

11. Some people are fulfilled when they are arguing or fighting; others like peace and cooperation.

12. Much healing of emotional illness results from loving and being loved.

13. Prejudice has sent many to an early grave and none of us is totally without some form of it.

14. Both a rickety church building on a creek bank up Buckhorn Creek and the Washington Cathedral in Washington, D.C. can be a place where people meet their God.

15. There are many roads to God and many roads to success. There are prophets out there who claim to have all the answers. Don't you believe it.

Part Five:

Stories From The Long Ago

—1—
Stories From The Long Ago

Street Cars And Trolley Cars

Public transportation in Louisville in the 1930's was in high gear. It had to be. Not many people had automobiles compared to today's scene. In no way did a youth have a vehicle of his own. It was unheard of. Many married couples with a family didn't either. We depended on trolley cars, trains, and buses to get from place to place. The trolley cars ran on certain main thoroughfares and were dependable. Not a speedy way to travel, not deluxe, but basic unhurried transportation. It cost three tokens for a quarter and a token could take you from one end of Louisville to another. One or two transfer slips were needed to transfer to other street cars but at no extra cost. Chestnut Street in Louisville had a short stubby trolley which took me from medical school to Preston Street. I transferred to the Preston Street trolley and went out to Eastern

Parkway turnaround and there caught a bus to Audubon Park where I lived. All the medical students had an unmistakable odor coming from their clothes and skin. To be exact, it was embalming fluid. We usually went to the rear of the trolley for reasons which are obvious.

Deep Water

At the Audubon Country Club swimming pool in Louisville I learned to swim one summer. I was ready to take my swimming test and prove to the lifeguards I could go to the deep end of the pool. Although I could swim well enough, I had never been in water over my head. I got ready to dive in the deep end of the pool, but I froze. Fear and uncertainty got me. I wouldn't dive in, I just stood there and looked into the water. Finally a buddy of mine came along behind me and shoved me in. I swam fine. If he hadn't done it I wonder how long it would have taken me to gather up the courage. After I did it, I knew I could. No more fear. A lot of truth here. A shove at the right time is all we need on many occasions.

Strep Throat

I had one strep throat after another when I was a kid. No penicillin, only salt water gargle. It took a week or ten days in bed with high fever to recover. Our family doctor didn't believe in food so long as you had a fever. I will never forget how hungry I would get until my fever broke and I could eat. I would eat about anything at that point. Finally Mom and Dad decided to go ahead and get my tonsils out. They knew I was worried about that so they didn't mention it to me until the very last minute. At the last moment they said that we were going to the doctor's office. When I was told what was forthcoming I had a panic attack. I had heard about a child who died during a tonsillectomy and I somehow knew I would not live through it. After an hour of panic I finally yielded and went peacefully to the death chamber. It was not a hospital.

I went to Dr. Anderson's office in the Breslen Building at Third and Broadway. It is now known as the Fincastle Building. I remember the strange sensation during the induction period of the anesthetic and then waking up feeling like I would die for sure. I finally was able to leave so I was put into a wheelchair and down the elevator I went. It was July and there was no air conditioning. It was terribly hot. I knew I would die before I got home but I didn't. For a week it felt like I had swallowed a bunch of razor blades. I recovered. I didn't think I would.

Bozo

I had a bulldog named Bozo. He wasn't good for much, but I loved him and he was a good fighter. He didn't keep away intruders; he just fought other dogs, one dog in particular. Three doors down was a dog named Pat, another bulldog. Bozo and Pat had it out regularly and they usually inflicted a lot of damage. Bozo would stay in his bed and lick his wounds for two to three weeks after a fight. Dogs didn't seem to fight if they were alone. If I showed up or if Jim or Ed Oehrle arrived on the scene, and the dogs saw us, they immediately started fighting. I suppose it was to prove to their master who was top dog. We devised various means to separate the dogs and stop the fight. Sometimes we were bitten in the process. The best way was to drop a wash tub down over one dog. You sure can't fight a wash tub.

Ferry Boats To Indiana

In the 1930's only a few cars and trucks were in Louisville compared to today. Only one bridge was available to carry the traffic to and from Indiana. The old K & I railroad bridge had only one lane going each way on either side of the railroad track but it seemed adequate. There was a ferry boat that made frequent trips from Louisville to Jeffersonville. It stopped near the site of the Second Street bridge. The ferry boat ride took a while but many preferred it rather than to go all the way to West Louisville and over to New Albany and then back to Jeffersonville. As a six year old boy I am sure I enjoyed the ride a lot more than my dad.

Audubon Park

A delight of my boyhood in Audubon Park was the day the Donaldson Bakery horse and wagon came through the park tempting us with the most delicious freshly baked goods with a marvelous aroma. The bakery man with a tray of goodies came to each door and Mom often yielded to my plea to buy some of that wonderful stuff. The ice cream truck would come in the evening with eskimo pies and chocolate covered ice cream bars. Then there was the ice wagon. Two to three times a week it made the rounds. You put in the front window of your home a card indicating the size of the chunk of ice you needed for your ice box and it would be delivered into your ice box as you had requested. Early in the morning, the milk man would bring your milk and leave it on your back porch in quart bottles, not plastic. You would leave empties for him to pick up. The only thing they delivered in those days that still is, is the daily newspaper.

Hot Stove

I was five years old at the time and one evening after taking my bath I climbed out of the tub and stood on the commode for Mom to dry me off. It was winter time and a gas stove was red hot and very near to the commode. I slipped on the wet top and fell across the stove. I can still feel the pain. The doctor was called and he gave instructions. I was greased with salve and wrapped up with gauze. It took a long time to recover. I don't have any scars and after this I dried off in another spot. Most lessons are learned the hard way.

Cess Pool Baseball

We played baseball in my backyard. Third base was a wooden board that was in the ground recessed a few inches.

I never knew exactly what its purpose was. One day a buddy slid into third base and he went through the wood board into a hole and disappeared all but his head and outstretched arms. What third base was, was the cap of our septic tank. Billy almost went somewhere he was not planning to go. We learned a lesson. Be wary of third base. We modified the playing field.

Fountaine-Ferry Park

Fountaine-Ferry Park was a little bit of heaven to Louisville kids. It was our one and only amusement park where about every exciting experience in the life of a kid could be had. There were ferris wheels, a roller coaster, all manner of rides, fun houses, spook houses. There was the merry-go-round, animals to ride, and a hundred games to play. At least once a year we went to Fountaine-Ferry Park. Often it was the school picnic. It seemed as if there were a million kids there and you stood in long lines to get on the rides, but it was worth it.

Daw Gone

Our neighbor in Audubon Park whose lot joined us in the back yard raised Airedale dogs in a kennel. We had nonstop barking and howling and yapping or so it seemed. It did get a little old at times. But you had to endure it. One day my dad, who used to make uncomplimentary remarks about the situation, got up and looked out back. The dogs were gone, everyone of them. We learned that they had been sold whereupon my dad exclaimed, "Well, I'll be daw-goned."

Haunted House In Paradise

Through the years I have made an occasional trip to Audubon Park to revel in nostalgia and touch base with some of my roots. Included in the itinerary would be a ride down Linnet Road to 3211 where I lived until I went away to college. The house was sold in 1948 and my parents moved to another part of Louisville. The house was built in 1927 or thereabouts and looks better today than it did then, I do believe. One reason is the presence of lovely trees and landscaping. The entire subdivision of Audubon Park is lovely for that very reason. The house is kept in excellent condition. That is also true of almost all the houses throughout the park. There is no part of Louisville that can compare to the beauty of Audubon Park during the Dogwood Festival. On one of my visits to my old home I got one of the shocks of my life. The place looked like an abandoned haunted house. So help me, the uncut grass was knee high or higher and the house needed painting and cleaning up in the worst way. Why should such a thing exist in the midst of such beauty? All the neighbors had kept up their property without exception. I made inquiry and found out to my dismay that a demented old lady lived in the house and was not about to let anyone come near her place or in her house. She was unreachable by friends or family and so the eyesore remained as it was for a long period of time. Finally, a clean up began. The old lady died and the house was sold and restored to its usual beauty and elegance. I took my mother by to see the house soon thereafter. We gathered the courage to go up to the door and knock. A lady came to the door, she was trusting and gracious and let us come in. We wanted to see our old home. What a treat!

Thanksgiving Day Hysteria

Hoosier hysteria is basketball. Fifty years ago in Louisville Thanksgiving Day hysteria was the annual Male-Manual football game at the Dupont Manual Stadium. During Thanksgiving week precious little was accomplished at the two schools other than to prepare for the game of games. If the team could win that game, it was a successful season, even if all the rest of the games were lost. Monday, Tuesday and Wednesday of

Thanksgiving week were the pep rally days at the Manual gym where I went to school. Our coach was Ray Baer and he was good at coaching, superb in building school spirit and a motivator second to none. During my three years at Manual (1939-1941) we managed to beat Male every year. In 1941 the score was Manual 40, Male 7. We had a national championship team and went on to win the title at Baton Rouge, Louisiana on New Year's Day. We played New Britton, Connecticut and won the game 28-20 and became the high school national football champions for the year. Billy Freeman, Clarence Sidebottom, and Johnny Meihaus were outstanding players, as I recall. Schools were segregated in those days, not only by race but by gender. Only white males were at Male and Manual and at St. Xavier. At Central High School in Louisville were black boys and girls. At Atherton Girl's high and Sacred Heart Academy were to be found the girls. It is all mixed up now, but I am not sure if it has helped the learning process. Culturally and socially I presume it was a wise change.

1937 Flood

I was 13 years old when the never to be forgotten big one hit Louisville. In Noah's day it rained 40 days and 40 nights. In Louisville it rained every day for 30 days in the month of January. The creeks and river rose and the Ohio River became the instrument of death and destruction. Louisville, Jeffersonville, and New Albany were all the victims of the rising muddy waters. Many residents left the area for shelter away from the flood. My family tried to leave but couldn't. We went to the 10th Street Railroad Station but the last train north to Chicago (the Monon) had just departed and we had to go home and endure the privations. We were in south Louisville, not under flood water. But no utilities were available for over a month. No gas, electricity, and no water. Candles and flashlight batteries were all sold out. Kerosene was hard to find. We heated our house with coal, so we were warm. We caught rain water to drink and for cooking. We went to bed when it got dark. We had enough to eat.

There was a lot of hardship and suffering and loss for many. Downtown Louisville was a mess. A bellhop caught a fish in the lobby of the Brown Hotel. Typhoid shots were given at Prestonia School. Refugees were put up in shelters in many areas. It was a devastating disaster that required a long time for recovery. It was rumored in Louisville that Jeffersonville never would come out of it, but of course, she did as everyone else did. If it rains for a steady week in Louisville anyone over 60 gets nervous.

Grandma Cauble

She was little but mighty. I can still see her in the backyard at her Pekin, Indiana, home pointing her finger at one of the grandchildren and giving out admonitions to mend their ways. In many ways she ruled the roost and dear grandpa didn't object at all. He loved her dearly and gave her plenty of rope.

She was the mother of five children and they were reared in the "nurture and admonition of the Lord." My mother was the oldest and got the message loud and clear and passed it on to me. I have received the word but now have been obliged to mend and modify some of my indoctrinated convictions as I have been exposed to the real world. My children have likewise come to their own religious convictions based upon their exposure to the world of ideas and people.

One day I stepped on a rusty nail in the chicken house while gathering eggs. It went deep into my foot. We were discussing the next step which included the possibility of a visit to Doc Green's office in Pekin to get a tetanus shot. At this point grandma exclaimed that the shot was not necessary. I was delighted. She got a piece of fat bacon, put it into my shoe, and I kept it in place for the next two to three days. I didn't get tetanus but I sure had a dandy exposure.

Grandma was fond of Doc Green as were many Pekin folk. He was not known for his neat and attractive office exactly. Matter of fact, it was a mess according to grandma. I have heard this story many times over. One day grandma was there to pick up some medicine and doc couldn't find it. He fumbled around a bit in his search and suddenly fell backwards into a big cardboard box. She declares he virtually disappeared and all she could see was his feet and hands and the top of his head. She was able to extricate him after considerable effort. Doc's office still stands to this day in Pekin, a silent reminder of the good ole days when doctors came to the house and charged reasonable fees.

One Sunday grandma was not well and could not go to church. For some reason I stayed home with her. Bozo, my beloved bulldog, was there too. Came church time and grandma thought we ought to have church. And so we did. We had a song, Bible reading and prayers. Then the Lord's supper. We got a cracker for the bread and some grape juice. After the service, Bozo was sniffing the cracker and obviously wished not to be left out of the communion service. I asked grandma what she thought about giving the cracker to the dog. She wasn't prepared for this and had to ponder the situation for a time. Finally she said that she didn't think the Lord would mind and for me to go ahead and give it to Bozo. I did. I'm sure he was appreciative.

Grandma was a lover of flowers and had a green thumb if anybody did. She had a back porch with window panes on two sides which allowed light and warmth in the winter time. In this wonderful area she had plants all over the place as well as ferns. Begonias were in abundance and beautiful. Bougainvillea was a delight of color. There were lilies in season, a lemon tree and an orange tree that bore fruit. She loved her plants and I think they loved her.

Eventually grandma got Parkinson's Disease and toward the end dementia took its toll. She broke first one hip and then the other, had prostheses inserted each time at Norton Infirmary in Louisville. She didn't give up. She was a fighter. Grandpa and Anna Elliott tenderly took care of her until it was too much. To the Williams Nursing Home she went in Salem. She talked about heaven often and finally one day she made her journey where she wanted to go.

Kelly On The Flag Pole

A boyhood memory I shall never forget was seeing a guy named Kelly standing on a disc on top of a flagpole on top of a building in downtown Louisville, Kentucky. Unbelievable but true. It was high enough so that a fall would be certain death. He stood on a metal disc about plate size and there were no securing ropes or straps. He didn't come down for a thing. Food and drink was sent up and how he managed his bowels and bladder, I don't know. He was there three days and three nights. People stood on the street and gawked at him in disbelief. He made a living this way going from city to city. He made it through without a mishap and went on to his next assignment.

One wonders what kind of a human would do this. A dare devil? An exhibitionist? A crazy man? Maybe a little bit of all three. Suffice it to say, the field of dare devils is not overcrowded, and I suspect he earned whatever he made in the process.

Not many of us would qualify for flagpole standing for obvious reasons. Yet, all of us, at least most of us, do enjoy getting attention in one way or another. Children have their way and adults have theirs. Methods are different but motivation is the same.

The attention getters who use their tongue non-stop can be a bore. The entertainers who are good get our attention. The super stars in Hollywood, in the pulpit, in the classroom, in the courtroom, on the political circuit, get our attention. There are plenty of people who get our attention who pose a real problem to society. These are the criminals and the law breakers in general. And there are others who demand our attention. The chronically ill people get lots of attention from the health care system. Those who are dependent on others or on society receive lots of attention.

Let's give three cheers for the masses out there who do their job, obey the law, and don't receive any trophies, accolades or newspaper coverage. Because of them we can have a decent world. Yes, a bouquet to the average guy or gal.

Tidbits For All Of Us

1. The telephone is a blessing and a curse. Life is like that. Blessings can turn into curses quickly and without warning.
2. AIDS threatens the existence of the human race. Maybe it can be its salvation. A common enemy is known to bring people together rather than separate them.
3. When someone of influence and power is on our side, we regard them as great people. When against us, we are inclined to say they are incompetent or dreadfully mistaken.
4. It's a good thing our maker placed our eyes back into our skull a distance, otherwise, we'd all be blind by the time we were adults.
5. A wood fire is warm, cozy company and a welcome friend on a cold, snowy night.
6. The solo flight can be scary and sometimes fatal, but if successful, brings growth, encouragement, and confidence.
7. If you complain excessively and unnecessarily, you may not be heard if and when you really get sick.

8. Don't become unduly depressed about the mistakes you inevitably will make, only God is perfect.

9. To walk a tightrope is uncertain and dangerous, but if we get across it is exhilarating. The Amish buggies may be slow, but the insurance bills are slower.

10. Credit cards are great for convenience but booby traps for credit.

11. Knowing all the facts doesn't necessarily make decision making easier.

12. Blessed are those who have their health and enough to eat.

13. Fortunate are we if we have a working partner that fits.

14. Frugality we don't admire, but most of us could use a small dose of it when approaching the mall.

15. We especially admire the person who struggles against tremendous odds and makes the grade.

16. Clean up your act, or someone else may try.

17. We look forward to family reunions but it is good to go home again.

18. Our maker made the opposite sex irresistable for the ongoing of the species and for pleasure, but the AIDS virus tells us we must call upon discipline if the race is to go on and our pleasures not be followed by disaster.

19. Most of us have a few eccentricities and many of us have a few crazies. Be guarded in harping on the other guy's behavior, you are likely to be a bit bizarre yourself.

20. To live with dignity is essential and to die with dignity is too.

21. We no longer fight at Gettysburg, we fight in the courtroom.

22. Prisons are unhappy places. One doesn't have to be behind bars to be in prison. Many people are locked up in situations from which they have no escape.

23. Olympic gold with humility makes a neat package.

24. Beware of criticizing the murderer, if the conditions were similar you might do the same.

25. Americans can go to the moon and back but we can't make a flashlight that works very long.

26. It is easy to worship our athletic and military heroes, and that's okay. But there are many other heroes out there who need recognition too.

27. The creator and designer of all that is, gave each organism a means of defense and offense. The rattlesnake has its deadly venom while mankind has its guns. Sometimes it appears that snakes will be here after men have destroyed themselves.

28. The one who loves his work is a happy person.

29. Prejudice and ignorance bring on much turmoil and unhappiness. We are all infected to some degree.

30. A true friend is a godsend.

31. Little towns in America are often in a state of decay, and when they go we have nothing to adequately replace them.

32. When your situation in life is intolerable, dementia then can be a blessing.

33. The first time you want to mountain climb, don't take on Mount Everest, try the Borden Knobs.

34. Only a few can sing during adversity.

35. We complain about driving coast to coast and with good reason, but it's a breeze compared to the covered wagon our ancestors used.

36. The size of the affluent's bank account is not the important thing. What is done with the money is.

37. When I was a medical officer on a navy ship during the Korean War, dogs and cats were not allowed on shipboard. Now females are allowed on board. That may solve some problems, but it creates a number of others. It is said that after two months at sea, any female looks like Miss America.

38. The gourmet meal is one in which you can't recognize a thing you have eaten. There never is an abundance, and good thing, it doesn't usually taste all that good.

39. Thank God for people of thought and talent who have written it down before they died. We are the benefactors.

40. Drive to an overlook in the mountains and the view is gorgeous. But all around you are other people, and rock and roll music, and dogs doing their business on car wheels. It sort of robs you of the joy. But climb a mountain alone or with your buddy and when you reach the summit, it is all yours to enjoy, no other people, no exhaust fumes, no dog barking, just you and God and the beautiful world. The struggle was worth it.

41. We affluent like our second homes on the lake and our swimming pools in the back yard. Maybe if we had the guts to shunt our surplus into *Habitat for Humanity* it would make the world a better place.

42. We all love recognition for our successes and on occasion have been known to brag about them, but for some reason we like to read about tragedies and misfortunes of others, not their successes. Interesting, isn't it?

43. If the money and energies we Americans expend suing each other could be directed toward fighting the drug war, the nation would be infinitely better off.

44. Perhaps we shouldn't see ourselves as others see us. Maybe we couldn't accept the truth.

45. And finally, as my Dad used to say when I was a kid, "Good night, sleep tight and don't let the bed bugs bite."

If you would like to purchase a copy of *Tidbits For Young Doctors,* please send your order to:

Donald L. Martin, M.D.
Box 289
Salem, IN 47167

Send check for $10.00 plus $3.00 for postage and handling. Tax is included.